Hip Dysplasia Surgery: Birth to Adulthood

Guest Editors

GEORGE J. HAIDUKEWYCH, MD
ERNEST L. SINK, MD

ORTHOPEDIC CLINICS OF NORTH AMERICA

www.orthopedic.theclinics.com

July 2012 • Volume 43 • Number 3

SAUNDERS an imprint of ELSEVIER, Inc.

W.B. SAUNDERS COMPANY
A Division of Elsevier Inc.

1600 John F. Kennedy Blvd. • Suite 1800 • Philadelphia, PA 19103-2899.

http://www.orthopedic.theclinics.com

ORTHOPEDIC CLINICS OF NORTH AMERICA Volume 43, Number 3
July 2012 ISSN 0030-5898, ISBN-13: 978-1-4557-3906-6

Editor: David Parsons

Orthopedic Clinics of North America (ISSN 0030-5898) is published quarterly by Elsevier Inc., 360 Park Avenue South, New York, NY 10010-1710. Months of issue are January, April, July, and October. Business and Editorial Offices: 1600 John F. Kennedy Blvd., Suite 1800, Philadelphia, PA 19103-2899. Customer Service Office: 3251 Riverport Lane, Maryland Heights, MO 63043. Periodicals postage paid at New York, NY and additional mailing offices. Subscription prices are $293.00 per year for (US individuals), $554.00 per year for (US institutions), $347.00 per year (Canadian individuals), $664.00 per year (Canadian institutions), $427.00 per year (international individuals), $664.00 per year (international institutions), $144.00 per year (US students), $208.00 per year (Canadian and international students). Foreign air speed delivery is included in all *Clinics* subscription prices. All prices are subject to change without notice. **POSTMASTER:** Send change of address to *Orthopedic Clinics of North America*, **Elsevier Health Sciences Division, Subscription Customer Service, 3251 Riverport Lane, Maryland Heights, MO 63043. Customer Service (orders, claims, online, change of address): Elsevier Health Sciences Division, Subscription Customer Service, 3251 Riverport Lane, Maryland Heights, MO 63043. Tel: 1-800-654-2452 (U.S. and Canada); 314-447-8871 (outside U.S. and Canada). Fax: 314-447-8029. E-mail: journalscustomerservice-usa@elsevier. com (for print support); journalsonlinesupport-usa@elsevier.com (for online support).**

Reprints. For copies of 100 or more, of articles in this publication, please contact the Commercial Reprints Department, Elsevier Inc., 360 Park Avenue South, New York, NY 10010-1710. Tel.: 212-633-3812; Fax: 212-462-1935; E-mail: reprints@elsevier. com.

Orthopedic Clinics of North America is covered in *MEDLINE/PubMed* (*Index Medicus*), *Cinahl, Excerpta Medica, and Cumulative Index to Nursing and Allied Health Literature.*

Printed and bound by CPI Group (UK) Ltd, Croydon, CR0 4YY

Transferred to digital print 2012

Contributors

GUEST EDITORS

GEORGE J. HAIDUKEWYCH, MD
Professor, Director of Orthopedic Trauma, Director, Complex Adult Reconstructive Service, Orlando Regional Medical Center, University of Central Florida, Orlando, Florida

ERNEST L. SINK, MD
Associate Professor, Weil Cornell Medical School; Center for Hip Pain and Preservation, Hospital for Special Surgery, New York, New York

AUTHORS

DANIEL J. BERRY, MD
LZ Gund Professor and Chairman, Department of Orthopedic Surgery, Mayo Clinic, Rochester, Minnesota

BERND BITTERSOHL, MD
Department of Orthopedic Surgery, Rady Children's Hospital San Diego, San Diego, California

PABLO CASTANEDA, MD
Shriners Hospital, Mexico, Distrito Federal, Mexico

NICHOLAS M.P. CLARKE, ChM, FRCS
Professor, Southampton General Hospital, Southampton, United Kingdom

MICHELE R. DAPUZZO, MD
Resident, Department of Orthopaedic Surgery, University of Virginia, Charlottesville, Virginia

GEORGE J. HAIDUKEWYCH, MD
Professor, Director of Orthopedic Trauma, Director, Complex Adult Reconstructive Service, Orlando Regional Medical Center, University of Central Florida, Orlando, Florida

HARISH S. HOSALKAR, MD
Department of Orthopedic Surgery, Rady Children's Hospital San Diego, San Diego, California

SIMON P. KELLEY, MBChB, FRCS (Tr and Orth)
Division of Orthopaedic Surgery, The Hospital for Sick Children, Toronto, Canada

YOUNG-JO KIM, MD, PhD
Associate Professor, Department of Orthopedics, Harvard Medical School; Director, Adolescent and Young Adult Hip Program, Department of Orthopedics, Children's Hospital Boston, Boston, Massachusetts

CARA BETH LEE, MD
Orthopedic Surgeon, Center for Hip Preservation, Department of Orthopedics, Virginia Mason Medical Center, Seattle, Washington

DROR PALEY, MD, FRCSC
Director, Paley Advanced Limb Lengthening Institute, St Mary's Hospital, West Palm Beach, Florida; Adjunct Professor, University of Toronto School of Medicine, Toronto, Canada; Professor, University of Vermont School of Medicine, Burlington, Vermont

KEVIN I. PERRY, MD
Department of Orthopedic Surgery, Mayo Clinic, Rochester, Minnesota

JEFFREY PETRIE, MD
Orlando Health Orthopedic Residency, Orlando, Florida

CHARLES T. PRICE, MD
Arnold Palmer Hospital for Children; Professor of Orthopedic Surgery, University of Central Florida College of Medicine, Orlando, Florida

BRANDON A. RAMO, MD
Arnold Palmer Hospital for Children, Orlando,
Florida

ADAM A. SASSOON, MD
Department of Orthopedic Surgery, Mayo
Clinic, Rochester, Minnesota

M. WADE SHRADER, MD
Clinical Assistant Professor of Orthopaedic
Surgery, University of Arizona College of
Medicine; Pediatric Orthopaedic Surgeon and
Director of Research, Center for Pediatrics
Orthopaedic Surgery, Phoenix Children's
Hospital, Phoenix, Arizona

RAFAEL J. SIERRA, MD
Associate Professor, Department of
Orthopaedic Surgery, Mayo Clinic, Rochester,
Minnesota

ERNEST L. SINK, MD
Associate Professor, Weil Cornell Medical
School; Center for Hip Pain and Preservation,
Hospital for Special Surgery, New York,
New York

LISA M. TIBOR, MD
Center for Hip Pain and Preservation, Hospital
for Special Surgery, New York, New York

ROBERT T. TROUSDALE, MD
Professor, Department of Orthopedic Surgery,
Mayo Clinic, Rochester, Minnesota

JOHN H. WEDGE, O.C., MD, FRCSC
Division of Orthopaedic Surgery, The Hospital
for Sick Children, Toronto, Canada

DENNIS R. WENGER, MD
Department of Orthopedic Surgery, Rady
Children's Hospital San Diego/University of
California, San Diego, San Diego, California

Contents

well as the joint orientation angle (medial proximal femoral angle) and the neck shaft angle. Femoral osteotomy can be performed on its own or in combination with greater trochanteric transfer. The location of the lesser trochanter must also be considered. Other considerations are the shape of the femoral head, the congruity of the joint, and the presence of acetabular dysplasia. Optimizing the anatomy of the hip joint offers the longest-term joint preservation and normalization of function.

a significant portion of the component uncovered, the alternatives include acetabular augmentation with bone autograft, intentional high placement of the component, or medialization of the component with or without medial wall osteotomy. Uncemented sockets have provided promising midterm results with supplemental bone augmentation and are the authors' preferred method of treatment for hips with moderate dysplasia and anterolateral acetabular bone deficiency.

ORTHOPEDIC CLINICS OF NORTH AMERICA

Prevention of Hip Dysplasia in Children and Adults

Charles T. Price, MD[a],*, Brandon A. Ramo, MD[b]

KEYWORDS

- Hip dysplasia • Neonatal hip instability • Adult hip dysplasia • Hip • Dysplasia • DDH

KEY POINTS

- Current efforts for prevention of hip dysplasia are primarily focused on early detection and early intervention to avoid long-term consequences of neglected hip dysplasia.
- Better prevention may be possible by decreasing postnatal environmental factors that influence the development of hip dysplasia.
- Methods of prevention have focused on neonatal hip instability although 90% of adult acetabular dysplasia is unrecognized during childhood.

Early diagnosis and early treatment of congenital dislocation of the hip are now possible. The next great challenge is the prevention of this serious and disabling condition.
—Robert B. Salter, Alexander Gibson Memorial Address, University of Manitoba, October 27, 1967

INTRODUCTION

A discussion of the prevention of developmental dysplasia of the hip (DDH) in children and adults must first define the term, *disease prevention*. This simple point is important because current approaches often focus on early diagnosis and treatment to prevent adverse long-term effects. In contrast, true disease prevention seeks to eradicate the disease so that the treating physicians never encounter the problem. An obvious example is the eradication of smallpox or elimination of polio in Western countries. This article considers opportunities for early detection in addition to possibilities for true prevention of hip dysplasia. A brief review of the natural history, prevalence, and etiology is used to frame the discussion of prevention.

THE NATURAL HISTORY OF DEVELOPMENTAL DYSPLASIA OF THE HIP

Perhaps the best description of the long-term effects of untreated hip dysplasia is that of Canadian Indians observed in Manitoba by Corrigan and Segal[1] in the 1940s:

> The senior author first visited Island Lake in the summer of 1940 to attend as the government doctor at the annual treaty payments. He had never seen so many cripples all gathered together in one place outside of a hospital. It was easy to see that a large number of the cripples were cases of congenital dislocation of the hip, some bilateral, some unilateral. Some crawled on their hands and knees, some hopped about like clowns, others waddled like ducks. All accepted with typical stoicism their misfortune as life's lot. They knew no different. Nature had exacted another toll.[1]

There are few scientific reports of the long-term natural history of untreated DDH. Wedge and Wasylenko[2] provided some insight in a study of 54 adults with unilateral or bilateral dysplasia or

[a] Department of Orthopedic Surgery, Orlando Health, 1222 Orange Avenue, Orlando, FL 32806, USA; [b] Arnold Palmer Hospital for Children, 83 West Columbia Street, Orlando, FL 32806, USA
* Corresponding author.
E-mail address: charles.price@orlandohealth.com

Orthop Clin N Am 43 (2012) 269–279
doi:10.1016/j.ocl.2012.05.001
0030-5898/12/$ – see front matter © 2012 Elsevier Inc. All rights reserved.

frank dislocation. These investigators reported that a false acetabulum correlated with lower modified Harris hip scores because of degenerative changes of the femoral head and false acetabulum. Patients with dysplasia and subluxation had more disability and earlier onset of osteoarthritis than those with frank dislocations (**Fig. 1**). Overall, the investigators reported that 60% of the hips had poor outcomes. This high rate of poor outcomes might be assumed to increase with longer-term follow-up because half the patients were younger than age fifty at time of follow-up. There is no longer any doubt that treatment improves the natural history of DDH, but untreated hip dislocations still occur in remote regions of countries, such as Mexico, Ecuador, and Iraq.

DISEASE PREVALENCE, SCOPE, AND IMPORTANCE

Hip dysplasia affects approximately 1% to 3% of newborn infants although 4% to 6% may be affected if milder forms are included.[3,4] The combined total of all heart anomalies exceeds the incidence of hip dysplasia, but the specific diagnosis of hip instability is the single most common abnormality in newborn infants.[5,6] Approximately 2 per 1000 (0.2%) infants have frank hip dislocation that can be detected at the time of newborn examination.[3,7] In addition, ultrasound studies have demonstrated dynamic hip instability and/or ultrasonographic hip dysplasia in 5% to 15% of all newborns.[8,9] Approximately 80% of mild cases of hip instability resolve spontaneously,[10] but evaluation or treatment is recommended for 2% to 3% of all children because of concerns regarding hip dysplasia.[7,11,12] Based on the number of new births in the United States each year, it is estimated that approximately 100,000 infants in this country undergo additional evaluation for or treatment of hip dysplasia each year. Although ultrasound screening has been criticized as overly sensitive, it may provide some insight into cases of predisposition to adult hip problems because 90% of adult hip dysplasia is undetected by clinical screening.[13] Thus, the true prevalence of infantile hip dysplasia is difficult to assess and depends in part on the definition of dysplasia and the population reported.

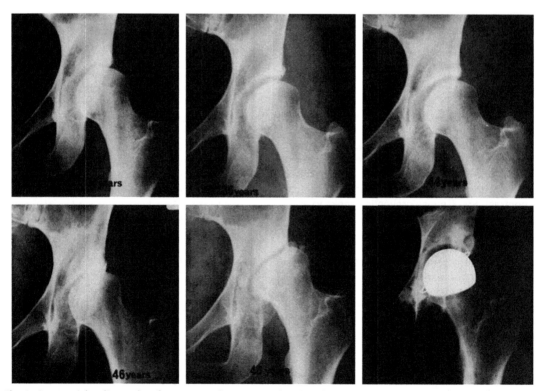

Fig. 1. Sequential radiographs of a woman who presented with mild hip pain and subluxation at 26 years of age (top left panel). Twenty years later she was disabled (bottom left panel) and subsequently required resurfacing arthroplasty (bottom right panel). (*From* Wedge JH, Wasylenko MJ. The natural history of congenital disease of the hip. J Bone Joint Surg Br 1979;61(3):334-8. *Reproduced* with permission and copyright © of the British Editorial Society of Bone and Joint Surgery.)

In the adult population, hip dysplasia is a substantial contributor to the development of hip arthritis.[13] Although primary osteoarthritis has been previously been identified as the most common cause of hip arthritis, this concept has been challenged by studies reporting a high prevalence of pre-existing hip deformity, such as acetabular dysplasia, as well as the pistol-grip deformity associated with slipped capital femoral epiphysis or femoroacetabular impingement.[14–16] Solomon[15] performed a clinical and radiographic analysis combined with postmortem examination of 327 cases of osteoarthritis of the hip. He identified acetabular dysplasia in 20%, with a male:female ratio of 1:10. In a radiographic study of primary osteoarthritis, Harris[14] estimated that 40% of cases were caused by underlying hip dysplasia. Harris also noted the preponderance of women with acetabular dysplasia. Hoaglund and Steinbach[16] summarized several historical articles, concluding that hip dysplasia accounts for approximately 10% of osteoarthritis of the hip. Using Hoaglund's more conservative estimate of 10% of cases of osteoarthritis attributable to hip dysplasia translates to approximately 25,000 total hip replacements (THRs) a year in the United States as a result of hip dysplasia.

Hip dysplasia plays an even greater role in the need for THRs in young people. Engsaeter, et al[13] in Norway reported that hip dysplasia is the origin of arthritis, requiring THR for approximately 20% of people younger than 40 years of age, and that 87% of those patients are women. In this study, 92% of patients with dysplasia requiring THR were undetected during childhood even though a national program for screening had been implemented in 1967. The Norwegian registry data also indicate that patients with neonatal hip instability (NHI) had a 2.6-times increased risk of early THR compared with children without NHI, although after treatment of NHI, numbers yield a low overall risk for THR before age 40. Although the data from Norway are useful, it is difficult to estimate the prevalence of unrecognized hip dysplasia in North America. If certain assumptions are made, then approximately 350,000 adults in the United States older than 40 are at risk for early hip arthritis because of dysplasia.[16,17] This estimate is based on the prevalence of osteoarthritis of the hip in Western countries combined with the estimated rate of dysplasia as a cause of osteoarthritis. By age 40, 1.3% of the population has osteoarthritis of the hip. This percentage rises to 14% after age 85 (**Fig. 2**).[17] The prevalence of hip arthritis for the entire adult population is 3% to 8%.[16,17] When these numbers are applied to the 140 million adults

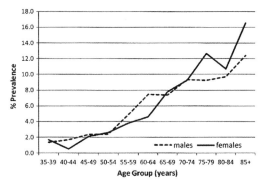

Fig. 2. Graph showing prevalence of radiographic hip osteoarthritis by age and gender. (*From* Dagenais S, Garbedian S, Wai EK. Systematic review of the prevalence of radiographic primary hip osteoarthritis. Clin Orthop Relat Res 2009;467:623–7; with permission.)

older than 40 in the United States,[18] and 10% of the hip arthritis is caused by dysplasia, then approximately 350,000 adults older than 40 are at risk for early hip arthritis because of dysplasia.[17]

To represent the spectrum of hip dysplasia, it may be advisable to distinguish between NHI and acetabular dysplasia that becomes evident later in life.[19] Perhaps the etiologies are different or perhaps the adult type of hip dysplasia was stable but undetectable during infancy. If prevention of NHI and adult acetabular dysplasia is possible, then the neonatal period is the logical time for preventive measures. To consider prevention, the etiology of hip dysplasia may provide an understanding of possible interventions to reduce the burden of disease for this common condition.

ETIOLOGY OF HIP DYSPLASIA

The role of inheritance in DDH is well known but hormonal and mechanical factors also affect the risk of NHI.[20] Inheritance may predispose infants to the adverse influence of hormonal or mechanical factors. Thus, the etiology is multifactorial but there is a 12-fold increase in risk for first-degree relatives.[20] If one child has hip dysplasia, the risk increases to 6% for a second child. The child of a parent with hip dysplasia has a 12% risk of having dysplasia. The risk is 36% for subsequent children when there is an affected parent and an affected child.[21] DDH is 4 to 5 times more prevalent in girls than in boys.[22] Girls may be especially susceptible to the maternal hormones estrogen and relaxin, which contribute to ligamentous laxity with resultant instability of the hip in the neonatal period.[23,24]

There are also risk factors related to intrauterine mechanical pressure, including breech position, oligohydramnios, increased birthweight, prim parity, older maternal age, and postmaturity.[25] Leutekort and colleagues[26] reported that hip joint instability was present in 47% of breech position babies born vaginally with the knees extended, whereas hip instability was noted in only 8% of vaginally delivered breech infants whose knees were flexed. The protective effect of knee flexion, younger gestational age, and lower birthweight has also been observed in twin births.[27] Breech infants born by caesarian section have a lower incidence of DDH than breech infants born vaginally.[25,28] These findings suggest that stretching of the hip capsule or hamstring muscles in utero predispose to hip dislocation in the neonatal period.

Postnatal mechanical factors also affect the development of hip dislocation. Hip dislocation has been produced in experimental animals by immobilization of the hips or knees in extension, but sectioning of the hamstring or psoas muscles reduced the frequency of hip dislocation.[23,29,30] In the experimental using animal models, the incidence of hip dislocation was also increased by addition of maternal hormones that promote hip joint laxity, and the effect was greater in female than in male animals.[23,30]

Normal human infants have an average hip flexion contracture of 28°. The hip flexion contracture decreases to 19° at 6 weeks and 7° at 3 months of age.[31,32] Hip flexion contractures of 50° and knee flexion contractures of 35° have also been noted in otherwise healthy newborn infants.[33] These hip and knee contractures improve rapidly in the newborn period and gradually resolve after the assumption of upright posture.[32,33] Forcing the hips and knees into extension during the neonatal period may predispose the immature hip to become unstable. Several investigators have cautioned against extension of the hip during the neonatal period because of increased risk of hip subluxation, dislocation, or dysplasia.[29,32,34]

These warnings to avoid forced or sustained extension of the lower limbs are supported by many reports of traditional swaddling. A study of Canadian Indians reported a 10-fold increase in the incidence of hip dislocation in tribes that carry babies on a cradleboard with the hips strapped in an extended and adducted position.[34] A high incidence of hip dislocation was reported in Navajos who strapped their infants to a cradleboard (**Fig. 3**).[35] The incidence of complete dislocation in the Navajo decreased dramatically in the 1940s, however, when diapers were introduced for use instead of leaves to absorb excreta. It was concluded that diapers kept the hips slightly abducted and flexed even when strapped in the cradleboard.

A somewhat similar experience has been documented in Japan.[23] In 1975 a national program was initiated in Japan to avoid swaddling infants

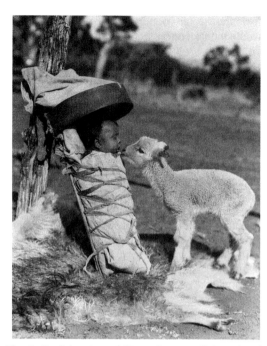

Fig. 3. Traditional swaddling using a cradleboard with the lower extremities held in adduction and extension. Cultures that use traditional swaddling have a high prevalence of hip dislocation. (© H. Armstrong Roberts.)

with the hips and knees in extension. Before that initiative, the incidence of infantile dislocation of the hip was 1.1% to 3.5%. After the public awareness campaign to eliminate traditional swaddling, the incidence of hip dysplasia in Japan dropped to less than 0.2%.[23] A significant relationship between swaddling and hip dysplasia has also been found in Turkey.[36] The frequency of hip dysplasia in Turkey was reduced through education for proper swaddling, but traditional swaddling is still the greatest risk factor for DDH in that country.[37] A systematic review of 11 epidemiologic articles supported a positive correlation between higher rates of DDH in swaddling cultures and concluded that DDH was adversely influenced by swaddling.[38] Further evidence that swaddling increases the risk of hip dysplasia is suggested by the observation of seasonal variations, with greater frequency of hip dislocations during the winter in colder climates.[39,40]

Swaddling is increasing in popularity in English-speaking countries. Demand for swaddling clothes increased 61% in Great Britain from 2010 to 2011.[41] In 2010, a survey indicated than 80% of infants in the United States are swaddled during the first few months of life because swaddling calms infants and improves sleep patterns and may decrease the risk of sudden infant death syndrome.[38,42] Mahan and Kasser[42] commented on the current swaddling trend and summarized the potential risk of hip dysplasia from improper swaddling. Mahan and Kasser cautioned, "For all infants who are swaddled, monitoring of the swaddling technique to ensure that their hips are allowed to flex and abduct in a safe position for hip development may lessen the risk of DDH."[42]

In contrast, hip dysplasia is rare in cultures that carry their infants with the hips abducted[34,43] (**Fig. 4**). The prevalence of osteoarthritis of the hip is also low in Hong Kong and Africa where these cultural practices are common.[16,17] In 1968, Robert Salter[39] observed, "...if the hips of all infants were protected by maintaining them in mild flexion and mild abduction during this [neonatal] period, it is possible that even if the congenitally dislocatable hip did in fact dislocate shortly after birth, it would not remain in the dislocated position and therefore would not become a persistent dislocation."[39]

Further support for perinatal and postnatal causes of hip dysplasia is found in ultrasonographic studies of hip development during later stages of gestation prior to delivery and also in preterm infants.[44,45] These studies indicate that the hip is well formed prior to birth. A study of fetal ultrasonography reported, "Prenatally, the mean α-angles were above the level that corresponds to a mature hip joint."[45] The acetabular

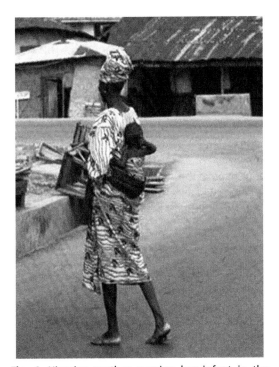

Fig. 4. Nigerian mother carrying her infant in the jockey position with the hips flexed and abducted. Cultures that carry their infants in this position have a low prevalence of hip dislocation.

roof angle decreased after birth in normal infants suggesting postnatal influences on developmental dysplasia. The same study evaluated preterm infants and noted that β angles were greater in term infants than in pre-term infants. Dissections in deceased newborn infants with hip dislocation have not always demonstrated primary acetabular dysplasia.[46] Thus, the concept of immature hip should be reconsidered with regards to anatomic development. These observations suggest that the hip may be more mature prior to birth and become more dysplastic around the time of birth. Therefore, although there are genetic influences on the development of hip dysplasia, perinatal and postnatal factors play an important role in the etiology of this condition. Thus, the best time for prevention of hip dysplasia is during birth and in the first few weeks of life.

PREVENTION BY EARLY DIAGNOSIS AND TREATMENT

Early diagnosis is important for prevention of long-term disability because early nonsurgical treatment with abduction devices decreases the frequency of surgery and improves long-term outcomes.[3,7,47] Various applications of newborn screening programs have been implemented in many regions of the world. Although some authorities have questioned the efficacy of any form of screening,[48] simple newborn examination and early treatment have reduced the burden of diseases where modern newborn care is widely practiced.[7,22,47] Screening is a topic unto itself. For a more thorough discussion, readers are referred to several recent summaries of the topic based on large literature reviews.[7,12,47,49–52]

In 2006, The United States Preventive Services Task Force concluded that there existed insufficient evidence to recommend routine screening of any sort (ultrasound or clinical) for DDH.[48] This conclusion was criticized by representatives of the Pediatric Orthopaedic Society of North America, who advised continuation of periodic clinical examination and selective ultrasound examination as recommended by the American Academy of Pediatrics.[22,47] The Canadian Task Force on Preventive Health Care determined that fair evidence existed to support serial clinical examination by trained clinicians for early detection of hip dysplasia. The Canadian Task Force recommended, however, against general or selective ultrasound screening citing the substantial "harms of labeling, repetitive investigations, unnecessary splinting and resource consumption associated with screening."[7] The American Academy of Pediatrics has supported serial clinical examination of the hips by a trained examiner as the current best method of screening for DDH with selective use of ultrasound.[22] For high-risk infants, the American Academy of Pediatrics recommends that infant girls born in the breech position have hip imaging either with ultrasound at 6 weeks of age or radiographs at 4 months of age. Hip imaging is optional in boys born in the breech position and in girls with a positive family history of DDH.

Among other Western countries, the National Health Service in the United Kingdom has a Newborn and Infant Physical Examination Programme, which, in March 2008, launched a standardized newborn examination to be performed within the first 72 hours of life and includes routine hip testing. There also exists a Standing Medical Advisory Committee that publishes updated guidelines on DDH screening that currently state all babies should be screened by physical examination within 24 hours of birth, prior to hospital discharge, at 6 weeks, between 6 and 9 months, and at walking age.[3]

A population-based study from Austria reported a small increase in costs with universal ultrasound screening but a 75% reduction in the number of surgical interventions compared with clinical screening alone.[53] One criticism of this study is that the comparisons were made in different time periods, with clinical screening alone from 1978 to 1982 and universal ultrasound screening from 1993 to 1997. Despite this study and other studies that have shown trends toward decreased rates of surgery for DDH, none has done so with convincing statistical significance compared with clinical screening by physical examination alone.[7,12,48,52,54]

Another major criticism of universal ultrasound screening is its high sensitivity, which leads to potential overtreatment. Some investigators have proposed a selective use of ultrasound screening only for hips presenting with risk factors of clinical instability, family history, breech presentation, and possibly postural foot deformities.[11] For those hips with mild ultrasonographic dysplasia, observation with sequential ultrasound studies can reduce the numbers of patients treated because approximately 50% of mild neonatal sonographic dysplasia spontaneously improves.[55] This selective approach to both ultrasound screening and treatment of sonographic dysplasia has been recommended by several investigators.[3,11,22,49,55,56]

Although the value of ultrasonography for detection of hip dysplasia is still debated and unclear, there is support for routine clinical examination in the newborn period followed by serial examination during the first year of life. The Canadian Task Force on Preventive Health care reported that prior to clinical screening, the operative rate for infant hip dysplasia was 1 to 2 per 1000, which was approximately the same as the overall treatment rate. After institution of routine clinical examination, approximately 5 to 20 cases per 1000 were treated for hip instability but the operative rate decreased to 0.2 to 0.7 per 1000. After the introduction of ultrasonography, approximately 40 to 50 cases per 1000 were treated for hip dysplasia but the operative rate remained 0.2 to 0.7 per 1000.[7]

An important aspect of clinical diagnosis is that clinicians must be properly trained and skilled in performance of the examination for hip instability. Instruction is often provided by videos, use of models, or bedside teaching during medical training. These methods are often unstructured or inconsistent. In an attempt to standardize and improve this educational process for health professionals, the Royal Children's Hospital in Melbourne, Australia, produced a 3-D animated instructional DVD. This teaching module has subsequently been validated with preinstruction and postinstruction testing 6 months and 2 years after instruction using the DVD module.[57] This teaching methodology has the potential to improve early diagnosis and treatment of hip dysplasia in many regions of the world where hip dysplasia is endemic and ultrasound screening is impractical because of limited resources.

WOULD HIGHER RATES OF TREATMENT PREVENT ADULT MORBIDITY FROM HIP DYSPLASIA?

Acetabular dysplasia as a risk factor for osteoarthritis in adults may not be detectable by clinical screening of infants.[13,19] It is unknown whether these late cases of dysplasia are residuals of infantile hip dysplasia or whether the condition develops during later periods of growth. One method of true prevention of the late dislocation or late dysplasia, however, might be to change the approach to early treatment. Sewell and Eastwood[49] suggested, "further research needs to establish whether early splintage of clinically stable but sonographically dysplastic hips affects future risk of late-presenting dysplasia/dislocation and osteoarthritis."[49] Dezateux and Rosendahl[58] proposed that trials assigning patients to treatment with abduction splinting or watchful waiting for infants in the borderline ultrasound categories might prove acceptable and might provide useful information about the natural history of hip dysplasia.

Rosendahl and colleagues[59] studied healthy newborn infants and reported that the mean α angle was 62.3 for girls and 65.3 for boys shortly after birth. Riad and colleagues[60] reported the development of 80 hips in 40 healthy babies who had ultrasound studies at birth and at 6 and 12 weeks to define normal progression of hip development. These investigators reported a mean α angle of 70.2° in the newborn period and 76.8° at 6 weeks of age. They also noted that an α angle of 65° or less was more than 2 SD from the mean at 6 weeks of age. Thus, it is questionable whether an α angle of 60° should be considered normal at any age beyond the first week of life. Regardless of these reports, observation is generally advised for Graf Type IIa (α angle 50°–60° prior to age 3 months) because there is poor correlation between ultrasound findings and subsequent radiographic measurements of dysplasia.[58,61,62] Also, an acetabular index of 30° at 1 year of age is frequently accepted as normal even though this is more than 2 SD from the mean.[55,63,64]

It is unknown whether earlier treatment of mild dysplasia would reduce the prevalence of acetabular dysplasia in adults. Proof that there is a correlation between ultrasonographic dysplasia and late osteoarthritis would require long-term follow-up and a prospective study may not be feasible. Efforts, such as those described in the following section, to prevent undetectable cases of hip dysplasia in late adolescence or adulthood may justify increased attention to mild forms of stable hip dysplasia during infancy.

TRUE PREVENTION DURING INFANCY

Early diagnosis and treatment of NHI has reduced the burden of disease in Western countries, but more than 90% of adult patients with acetabular dysplasia are overlooked or undetected by current methods of screening and treatment. Also, underdeveloped regions where neonatal hip dislocations are endemic rarely have resources to implement widespread screening programs, especially programs that rely on ultrasonography. Thus, true prevention should be inexpensive and easily applied. Two public health measures may warrant further evaluation. The first is swaddling education, and the second is the Klisic method of universal infant positioning during the neonatal period.

Swaddling education has reduced the prevalence of neonatal hip dislocations in Turkey and Japan and among Native Americans.[23,36,65] In Australia, there has been an increasing prevalence of DDH since 2003.[57] That increased frequency coincides with rising popularity of swaddling in that country. As a consequence, a national program to teach proper swaddling has been implemented. Similar public health education measures may reduce the burden of infantile hip dislocations in cultures that prefer tight swaddling of the lower extremities during the neonatal period. Educational measures may also be needed in Western countries where swaddling is becoming more popular.[42]

The Klisic method of prevention applied the advice of Salter to protect the hips of all infants by maintaining them in a position of mild flexion and mild abduction during the neonatal period.[39] Klisic and colleagues[66] outlined the distribution of baby packages free of charge to parents of every newborn child. This package included a wide diaper and a diaper cover to maintain hip abduction (Fig. 5). After free distribution of these baby packages for approximately a decade in

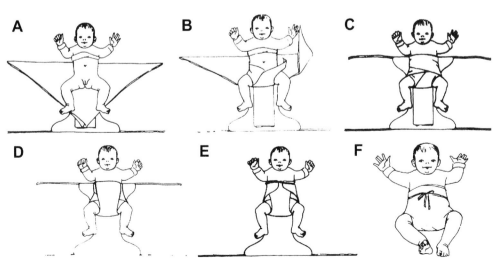

Fig. 5. (A–F) Klisic method of wide diapering with a hip package as illustrated in steps for parents of all newborn infants for prevention of hip dysplasia. (From Klisic P, Pajic D. Progress in the preventive approach to developmental dysplasia of the hip. J. Pediatr Orthop B 1993;2:108-11; with permission.)

Serbia, Klisic and colleagues reported a significant decrease in the prevalence of congenital dislocation of the hip. The rate of congenital dislocation of the hip fell from 1.3% in years prior to distribution of baby packages to a mean of 0.7% in the ensuing 4 years (**Fig. 6**). During this period, there was a 7-fold decrease in the number of surgical procedures for hip dislocation.[67]

Before Klisic and before implementation of screening programs, Judet and Gielis[68] proposed universal treatment of all subluxable hips. The investigators were frustrated by their inability to predict dysplasia or dislocations based on clinical examination or radiographic findings in the preultrasound era. Thus, Judet and Gielis introduced the concept of prevention rather than screening for the treatment of DDH. Judet and Gielis specifically proposed placing the legs in abduction of all newborns up to age 4 months and continuing this treatment longer in those with "malformations." They then proposed a radiograph of all children at 4 months to evaluate for residual dysplasia at which point hip abduction could be stopped if normal.

Klisic and colleagues[66] cited Judet and Gielis' comments when they put forth their method of universal prevention for DDH, which they termed, *triple prevention*. Klisic and colleagues' recommendations included (1) all newborns examined to identify any dislocations at birth; (2) regular wide diapering with hips in abduction of all presumably healthy hips (essentially all children) by means of soft abduction pants so as to direct possible cases of dysplasia toward normal development; and (3) re-examining all hips until walking age.

Soft abduction splints have also been used effectively for subluxable or dislocatable hips beginning in the newborn period.[55,64] They have successfully prevented more restrictive or more invasive interventions. Rosendahl and colleagues[55] conducted a blinded, randomized controlled trial of mildly dysplastic hips (α angle of 43°–49°). Patients were assigned either to immediate abduction treatment with a Frejka pillow or to observation. Hip ultrasound studies were performed at 6 weeks of age and radiographs at 2 years of age were used to determine the acetabular index. Among the immediately treated patients, all hips improved by 6 weeks of age and 8% required splinting after age 3 months. In the observation group, 81% had improved by age 6 weeks and 47% of patients required splinting after age 3 months. In both groups the average duration of treatment was 12 weeks and there were no differences in the acetabular indices. Thus, the final outcomes were equivalent in the immediately treated group and in the group that had sequential surveillance and selective treatment. This finding may have particular relevance for regions that lack resources for sequential surveillance. Also, the investigators noted, "...delaying treatment may limit an increasingly mobile child."[55]

Additional benefits of universal treatment may be to decrease the risk of late dislocation because late dislocation and dysplasia have been reported after normal ultrasound studies at 6 weeks of age. Imrie and colleagues[69] reported that 29% of breech infants developed hip dysplasia after a normal ultrasound and stable hip examination at 6 weeks of age.

One concern about universal treatment is the risk of avascular necrosis, but this has not been reported after treatment with soft abduction splints or pants applied in the newborn period to maintain physiologic hip positions.[64,67,68,70] A meta-analysis also reported that initiation of treatment after 2 months of age is associated with higher rates of avascular necrosis.[71]

As described in his original articles in the 1980s, Klisic's baby package cost less than $10 per child and was subsidized for some time by the government. Despite this seemingly high cost to developed nations with millions of births yearly, Klisic's form of universal prevention may be more cost effective than universal sonographic screening. More frequent treatment with simple devices may be an alternative to widespread diagnostic screening and targeted treatment of a few patients.

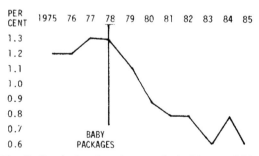

Fig. 6. Graph showing decrease in incidence of hip dislocation following distribution of hip packages for universal prevention of hip dysplasia in Serbia. (*From* Klisic P, Zivanovic V, Brdar R. Effects of triple prevention on CDH, stimulated by distribution of "baby packages". J Pediatr Orthop 1984;4:759–61; with permission.)

SUMMARY

Klisic and Pajic summarized the history of early diagnosis and treatment of hip dysplasia when they wrote,

> *Devising the preventive approach to developmental dysplasia of the hip (DDH) required*

much time.... Despite the 2400-year-old suggestion made by Hippocrates that children's hip dislocations are curable if treatment is started very early, the preventive approach was proposed by Roser only in 1879 [who] described early diagnosis in newborns and performed reduction by abduction... He also advocated early treatment by fixing babies' hips in abduction. However, surgeons did not readily accept these proposals, despite the good results shown by Froelich in 1906 and Le Damany in 1911. In 1927, Putti succeeded in interesting some orthopedic surgeons in the procedure by showing the results of early treatment. But the practical problem remained: ie, how to detect the DDH in patients at an early age. The turning point came in 1935 when pediatrician Ortolani introduced early detection of DDH by "early clinical search" shortly after a child's birth, instructing obstetricians, pediatricians, and midwives to perform the search. Rediscovering the diagnostic "segno della scatto," ie, reducible displacement, he popularized the prophylactic approach to DDH by early detection and treatment. Fifteen years later, another pediatrician, Palmen, organized systematic screening in nurseries by pediatricians.[72]

Since Klisic and Pajic wrote this in 1993, the use of ultrasound, albeit still controversial in some ways, has influenced the treatment and prevention of DDH. Klisic's attempts to universally prevent the disease may still be able to be incorporated into further efforts at disease prevention through education and the systematic trials of hip abduction pillows or braces similar to his wide-diaper diapering technique. The goal of prevention is to eradicate a disease so that it does not present to the physician. For DDH, this goal may be tenable.

REFERENCES

1. Corrigan C, Segal S. The incidence of dislocation of the hip at Island Lake, Manitoba. Can Med Assoc J 1950;62:535–40.
2. Wedge J, Wasylenko MJ. The natural history of congenital disease of the hip. J Bone Joint Surg 1979;61B:334–8.
3. Sewell M, Rosendahl K, Eastwood DM. Developmental dysplasia of the hip. BMJ 2009;339:b4454.
4. Roposch A, Liu LQ, Hefti F, et al. Standardized diagnostic criteria for developmental dysplasia of the hip in early infancy. Clin Orthop Relat Res 2011;469(12): 3451–61.
5. British Columbia Vital Statistics Agency. Health Status Registry Report: congenital anomalies, congenital defects, selected disabilities, British Columbia, Canada: Ministry of Health; 2005. p. 14–6.
6. Centers for Disease Control and Prevention. Surveillance for and comparison of birth defect prevalences in two geographic areas—United States, 1983–88. In: CDC surveillance summaries (March 19) MMWR 1993;42:(No. SS-1).
7. Patel H. Prevention Health Care, 2001 update: screening and management of developmental dysplasia of the hip in newborns. CMAJ 2001;164:1669–77.
8. Bialik V, Bialik GM, Blazer S, et al. Developmental dysplasia of the hip: a new approach to incidence. Pediatrics 1999;103:93–9.
9. Rosendahl K, Markestad T, Lie RT. Ultrasound screening for developmental dysplasia of the hip in the neonate: the effect on treatment rate and prevalence of late cases. Pediatrics 1994;94:47–52.
10. Barlow T. Early diagnosis and treatment of congenital dislocation of the hip. J Bone Joint Surg 1962; 44B:292–301.
11. Boree NR, Clarke NM. Ultrasound imaging and secondary screening for congenital dislocation of the hip. J Bone Joint Surg Br 1994;76:525–33.
12. Kocher M. Ultrasonographic screening for developmental dysplasia of the hip: an epidemiologic analysis (Part II). Am J Orthop 2001;30(1):19–24.
13. Engesaeter I, Lie SA, Lehmann TG, et al. Neonatal hip instability and risk of total hip replacement in young adulthood. Acta Orthop 2008;79:321–6.
14. Harris W. Etiology of osteoarthritis of the hip. Clin Orthop Relat Res 1986;213:20–33.
15. Solomon L. Patterns of osteoarthritis of the hip. J Bone Joint Surg 1976;58B(2):176–83.
16. Hoaglund FT, Steinbach LS. Primary osteoarthritis of the hip: etiology and epidemiology. J Am Acad Orthop Surg 2001;9:320–7.
17. Dagenais S, Garbedian S, Wai EK. Systematic review of the prevalence of radiographic primary hip osteoarthritis. Clin Orthop Relat Res 2009;467:623–7.
18. Howden LM. United States Census Bureau Age and sex composition: 2010. Washington: US Dept of Commerce; 2011.
19. Hvid I. Neonatal hip instability, developmental dysplasia of the acetabulum, and the risk of early osteoarthritis. Acta Orthop 2008;79(3):311–2.
20. Stevenson D, Mineau G, Kerber RA, et al. Familial predisposition to developemental dysplasia of the hip. J Pediatr Orthop 2009;29(5):463–6.
21. Wynn-Davies R. Acetabular dysplasia and familial joint laxity: two etiological factors in congenital dislocation of the hip: a review of 589 patients and their families. J Bone Joint Surg 1970;52B:704–16.
22. Clinical practice guideline: early detection of developmental dysplasia of the hip. Committee on Quality Improvement, Subcommittee on Developmental Dysplasia of the Hip. American Academy of Pediatrics. Pediatrics 2000;105(4):896–905.

23. Yamamuro T, Ishida K. Recent advances in the prevention, early diagnosis, and treatment of congenital dislocation of the hip in Japan. Clin Orthop Relat Res 1984;184:34–40.

24. MacLennan A. The role of relaxin in human reproduction. Clin Reprod Fertil 1983;2:77–95.

25. Chan A, McCaul KA, Cundy PJ, et al. Perinatal risk factors for developmental dysplasia of the hip. Arch Dis Child 1997;76:F94–100.

26. Lutekort M, Persson PH, Polberger S, et al. Hip joint instability in breech pregnancy. Acta Paediatr 1986; 75:860–3.

27. De Pellegrin M, Moharamzadeh D. Developmental dysplasia of the hip in twins: the importance of mechanical factors in the etiology of DDH. J Pediatr Orthop 2010;30(8):774–8.

28. Lowry C, Donoghue VB, O'Herlihy C, et al. Elective Caesarean section is associated with a reduction in developmental dysplasia of the hip in term breech infants. J Bone Joint Surg 2005;87B:984–5.

29. Suzuki S, Yamamuro T. The mechanical cause of congenital dislocation of the hip joint. Acta Orthop Scand 1993;64:303–4.

30. Wilkinson J, Carter C. Prime factors in the etiology of congenital dislocation of the hip. J Bone Joint Surg 1963;45B:268–83.

31. Haas S, Epps CH, Adams JP. Normal ranges of hip motion in the newborn. Clin Orthop Relat Res 1973; 91:114–8.

32. Coon V, Donato G, Houser C, et al. Normal ranges of hip motion in infants six weeks, three months, and six months of age. Clin Orthop Relat Res 1975;110:256–60.

33. Hoffer M. Joint motion limitation in newborns. Clin Orthop Relat Res 1980;148:94–6.

34. Salter R. Role of Innominate osteotomy in the treatment of congenital dislocation and subluxation of the hip in the older child. J Bone Joint Surg 1966;48A:413–39.

35. Pratt W, Freiberger RH, Arnold WD. Untreated congenital hip dysplasia in the Navajo. Clin Orthop Relat Res 1982;162:69–77.

36. Kutlu A, Memik R, Mutlu M, et al. Congenital dislocation of the ip and its relationship to swaddling used in Turkey. J Pediatr Orthop 1992;12: 598–602.

37. Dogruel H, Atalar H, Yavuz OY, et al. Clinical examination versus ultrasonography in detecting developmental dysplasia of the hip. Int Orthop 2008;32: 415–9.

38. van Sleuwen B, Engelberts AD, Boere-Boonekamp MM, et al. Swaddling: a systematic review. Pediatrics 2007; 120:e1097–106.

39. Salter R. Etiology, pathogenesis and possible prevention of congenital dislocation of the hip. Can Med Assoc J 1968;98:933–45.

40. Record R, Edwards JH. Environmental influences related to the etiology of congenital dislocation of the hip. Br J Prev Soc Med 1958;12:8–22.

41. Qureshi W. Swaddling baby is back in fashion. London: Reuters; 2011. Available at: http://www.reuters.com/article/2011/12/23/us-britain-swaddling-idUSTRE7BM0OB20111223. Accessed January 12, 2012.

42. Mahan S, Kasser JR. Does swaddling influence developmental dysplasia of the hip? Pediatrics 2008;121:177–8.

43. Hodgson A. Congenital dislocation of the hip. Br Med J 1961;2:647.

44. Gardiner H, Clarke NM, Dunn PM. A sonographic study of the morphology of the preterm neonatal hip. J Pediatr Orthop 1990;10:633–7.

45. Stiegler H, Hafner E, Schuchter K, et al. A sonographic study of prenatal hip development: from 34 weeks of gestation to 6 weeks of age. J Pediatr Orthop 2003;12B:365–8.

46. McKibben B. Anatomical factors in the stability of the hip joint in the newborn. J Bone Joint Surg 1970;52B:148–59.

47. Schwend R, Schoenecker P, Richards BS, et al. Screening the newborn for developmental dysplasia of the hip. J Pediatr Orthop 2007;27:607–10.

48. USPSTF. Screening for developmental dysplasia of the hip: recommendation statement. Pediatrics 2006;117:898–901.

49. Sewell M, Eastwood DM. Screening and treatment in developmental dysplasia of the hip—where do we go from here? Int Orthop 2011;35:1359–67.

50. Portinaro N, Pelillo F, Cerutti P. The role of ultrasonography in the diagnosis of developmental dysplasia of the hip. J Pediatr Orthop 2007;27(2): 247–50.

51. Shipman S, Helfand M, Moyer VA, et al. Screening for developmental dysplasia of the hip: a systematic literature review for the US Preventive Services Task Force. Pediatrics 2008;117: e557–76.

52. Woolacott N, Puhan MA, Steurer J, et al. Ultrasonography in screening for developmental dysplasia of the hip in newborns: a systematic review. Br Med J 2005;330(7505):1413.

53. Thaler MBR, Lair J, Krismer M, et al. Cost-effectiveness of universal ultrasound screening compared with clinical examination alone in the diagnosis and treatment of neonatal hip dysplasia in Austria. J Bone Joint Surg Br 2011;93(8):1126–30.

54. Shorter D, Hong T, Osborn Da. Screening programmes for developmental dysplasia of the hip in newborn infants. Cochrane Database Syst Rev 2011;(9):CD004595.

55. Rosendahl K, Dezateaux C, Fosse KR, et al. Immediate treatment versus sonographic surveillance for mild hip dysplasia in newborns. Pediatrics 2010; 125:e9–16.

56. Lowry C, Donoghue VB, Murphy JF. Auditing hip ultrasound screening of infants at increased risk of

developmental dysplasia of the hip. Arch Dis Child 2005;90:579–81.

57. Riley M, Halliday J. Developmental dysplasia of the hip. Victorian Birth Defects Bulletin, No. 7. Melbourne (Australia): Victorian Perinatal Data Collection Unit; 2009. p. 1–4.

58. Dezateaux C, Rosendahl K. Developmental dysplasia of the hip. Lancet 2007;369:1541–52.

59. Rosendahl K, Markestad T, Lie RT. Developmental dysplasia of the hip. A population-based comparison of ultrasound and clinical findings. Acta Paediatr 1996;85:64–9.

60. Riad J, Cundy P, Gent RJ, et al. Longitudinal study of normal hip development by ultrasound. J Pediatr Orthop 2005;25:5–9.

61. Dornacher D, Cakir B, Reichel H, et al. Early radiological outcome of ultrasound monitoring in infants with developmental dysplasia of the hips. J Pediatr Orthop 2010;19B:27–31.

62. Sucato D, Johnston CE, Birch JG, et al. Outcome of ultrasonographic hip abnormalities in clinically stable hips. J Pediatr Orthop 1999;19:754–9.

63. Tonnis D. Normal values of the hip joint for the evaluation of x-rays in children and adults. Clin Orthop Relat Res 1976;119:39–47.

64. Tredwell S, Davis LA. Prospective study of congenital dislocation of the hip. J Pediatr Orthop 1989;9:386–90.

65. Rabin D, Barnett CR, Arnold WD, et al. Untreated congenital hip disease: a study of the epidemiology, natural history, and social aspects of the disease in the Navajo population. Am J Public Health 1965; 55(2):1–44.

66. Klisic P, Rakic D, Pajic D. Triple prevention of congenital dislocation of the hip. J Pediatr Orthop 1984;4:759–61.

67. Klisic P, Zivanovic V, Brdar R. Effects of triple prevention of CDH, stimulated by distribution of "baby packages". J Pediatr Orthop 1988;8:9–11.

68. Judet J, Gielis L. Dépistage et traitement des luxations congénitales de la hanche. Acta Orthop Belg 1959;25:440–50.

69. Imrie M, Scott V, Stearns PH, et al. Is ultrasound screening for DDH in babies born breech sufficient? J Child Orthop 2010;4:3–8.

70. Mittelmeier H, Deimel D, Beger B. An ultrasound hip screening program – middle term results of flexion-abduction orthosis therapy. Z Orthop Ihre Grenzgeb 1998;136:513–8 [German].

71. Lehmann H, Hinton R, Morello P, et al. Developmental dysplasia of the hip practice guideline: technical report. Pediatrics 2000;105:e57.

72. Klisic P, Pajic D. Progress in the preventive approach to developmental dysplasia of the hip. J Pediatr Orthop B 1993;2B:108–11.

Strategies to Improve Nonoperative Childhood Management

Nicholas M.P. Clarke, ChM, FRCS[a],*, Pablo Castaneda, MD[b]

KEYWORDS

- Developmental dysplasia • Nonoperative management • Ultrasonography • Newborn

KEY POINTS

- Developmental dysplasia of the hip is the most common congenital defect in newborns,[1] with an estimated prevalence ranging from 1 to 30 per 1000 live births. Worldwide, 1 in 1000 children are born with a dislocated hip and 10 in 1000 children are born with hip instability or dysplasia.[1]
- The condition occurs with greater prevalence in certain cultures and is rarely observed in others. Cultural traditions, such as swaddling of the infant with the hips together in extension (as is customary in many native North American cultures), have been implicated as important causative factors in these groups.
- Approximately 80% of affected children are girls.
- The left hip is affected in about 60% of children, the right hip in 20%, and both hips in 20%. It is thought that the left hip is more frequently involved because it is adducted against the mother's lumbosacral spine in the most common intrauterine position (left occiput anterior); in that position, less cartilage is covered by the bone of the acetabulum and instability is, therefore, more likely to develop.
- The most widely accepted theory regarding the greater prevalence in girls speculates that girls may be affected more frequently because of the increased ligamentous laxity that transiently exists as the result of circulating maternal hormones and the additional effects of estrogen that are produced by the female infant's uterus,[2–4] although these findings have not been reproduced.

INTRODUCTION/OVERVIEW

The term, developmental dysplasia of the hip (DDH), has replaced the term, congenital dislocation of the hip, because it more accurately reflects the full spectrum of developmental abnormalities of the hip joint (**Fig. 1**).[5]

DDH or dislocation of the hip occurs more often in infants who present in the breech position, whether delivered vaginally or by cesarean section. The in utero knee extension of the infant in the breech position results in sustained hamstring forces regarding the hip with subsequent hip instability. Although breech presentation occurs in less than 5% of newborns, breech position has been noted in up to 32% of children with DDH.[6] Twice as many female infants as male infants present in the breech position, and 60% of breech presentations are noted in firstborn children. Firstborn children are affected twice as often as subsequent siblings presumably because of an unstretched uterus and tight abdominal structures, which may compress the uterine contents. Postural deformities and oligohydramnios are also associated with DDH.[3] The probability of having a child with DDH in at-risk families has been determined

[a] Southampton General Hospital, Tremona Road, Southampton, SO16 6YD, United Kingdom; [b] Shriner's Hospital, Sierra Nevada No 234, Lomas de Chapultepec, Mexico, DF 11000, Mexico
* Corresponding author.
E-mail address: ortho@soton.ac.uk

Orthop Clin N Am 43 (2012) 281–289
doi:10.1016/j.ocl.2012.05.002
0030-5898/12/$ – see front matter © 2012 Elsevier Inc. All rights reserved.

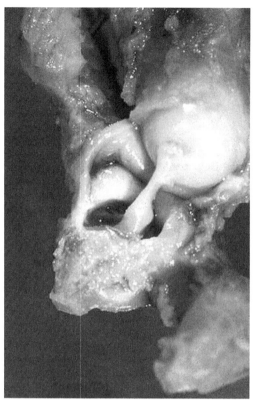

Fig. 1. Pathologic specimen of a congenitally dislocated hip in a breech baby. The labral deformity and infolded capsule are clearly seen.

by Wynne-Davies to be 6% if there are normal parents and one affected child; 12% if there is one affected parent but no prior affected child; and 36% if there is one affected parent and one affected child.

This condition can result in both subluxation and dislocation of the hip; a subluxated hip is one in which the femoral head is displaced from its normal position but still makes contact with the bony portion of the acetabulum. With a dislocated hip, there is no articular contact between the femoral head and the acetabulum.[7] This definition is based on radiographic findings and does not necessarily reflect the underlying pathoanatomical situation.

Acetabular dysplasia is characterized by a shallow or underdeveloped acetabulum. Dysplasia can exist with or without concomitant instability of the hip and, if untreated, may lead to a poorly located symptomatic hip. An unstable hip is one that is reduced in the acetabulum but can be provoked to subluxate or dislocate (ie, Barlow positive).[8,9] It should also be noted that there is a significant difference between clinical instability as found on examination and sonographic instability, which is only

found on dynamic sonogram testing; it can be difficult to distinguish some normal movements or clicks in healthy hips that have increased joint laxity, which makes it imperative that all newborns who have an equivocal physical examination be referred for further imaging, preferably with ultrasound. Estimates of the incidence range widely owing to the method used to detect the dysplasia, among other factors.[10,11] Early detection through neonatal screening along with the early initiation of treatment has lowered the rates of treatment-related complications, such as avascular necrosis of the femoral head and neck.[12,13] DDH is a leading cause of early arthritis. When the cost of the subsequent joint replacement surgery is considered, the impact from this condition is evident on any public health system.[14,15]

SCREENING

Neonatal screening for DDH can be performed by clinical examination[16] or ultrasonography.[17–20] Although neither of these tests carry any significant risk to patients, there is the possibility that universal ultrasound screening will detect several patients with abnormal findings that will resolve completely[1,8,10–20] (ie, a false-positive study); this, combined with the possibility of creating iatrogenic complications with the overtreatment of these possibly normal hips, has created some controversy over the efficacy of universal screening for hip dysplasia. Practices regarding screening vary according to country. In some German-speaking countries, it has been the custom to perform universal screening for many years; however, in the United States, there has been less enthusiasm for universal screening. In fact, although the current clinical practice guidelines of the American Academy of Pediatrics recommends screening for hip dysplasia,[21–23] the US Preventive Services Task Force recently concluded that "evidence is insufficient to recommend routine screening" for DDH because of the lack of clear scientific evidence favoring screening.[24] These conflicting statements make it difficult for the practicing clinician to make recommendations based on current opinion. A recent study by Mahan and colleagues[25] concludes that "the optimum strategy, associated with the highest probability of having a nonarthritic hip at the age of 60 years, was to screen all neonates for hip dysplasia with a physical examination and to use ultrasonography selectively for infants who are at high risk." This view is currently the view supported by the Pediatric Orthopedic Society of North America that recommends that all health care providers who are involved in the care of infants continue to follow the clinical practice guideline for early detection of DDH outlined by the American Academy of Pediatrics[26] and is the strategy that is about to be introduced in the United Kingdom.

Physical Examination

All newborn infants should be examined by a physician in the nursery. The history obtained at that first evaluation includes gestational age, presentation (breech vs vertex), type of delivery (cesarean vs vaginal), sex, birth order and family history of hip dislocation, ligamentous laxity, and myopathy. The baby should be relaxed and examined in a warm quiet environment with removal of the diaper. A general examination, beginning at the head, should be performed to detect conditions that are associated with an increased prevalence of DDH, such as torticollis, congenital dislocation of the knee or foot, lower-extremity deformities, and ligamentous laxity.[27,28]

The evaluation of the hip begins with the observation of both lower extremities for femoral shortening or asymmetry, although it should be noted that asymmetrical inguinal or thigh skin folds can be a normal finding. The Galeazzi or Allis sign is elicited by placing the child supine with the hips and knees flexed. Unequal knee heights suggest congenital femoral shortening or dislocation of the hip joint. Bilateral hip dislocation may be present and may not reveal asymmetry of femoral length or hip-joint motion. An infant with unilateral hip dislocation will eventually exhibit limited hip abduction on the affected side but perhaps not for several months. Each hip is examined individually with the opposite hip held in maximum abduction to lock the pelvis. Gentle, repetitive, passive motion of the hip joint will allow the detection of subtle instability. Soft tissue clicks felt while adducting or abducting the hip in the absence of other abnormal findings have been further evaluated with ultrasound and are considered benign.[29]

The Ortolani and Barlow tests are performed to evaluate hip stability. The infant must be examined in a relaxed state while positioned supine on a firm surface. Each hip is examined separately. To perform the Ortolani test on the left hip, the examiner's right hand gently grasps the left thigh with the middle or ring finger over the greater trochanter and the thumb over the lesser trochanter. The examiner's left hand is used to stabilize the infant's right hip in abduction. The examination is initiated by slowly and gently abducting the left thigh while simultaneously exerting an upward force on the left greater trochanter. Abduction of each hip should be symmetric. The sensation of a palpable clunk when the Ortolani maneuver is performed represents mechanical reduction of the femoral head into the confines of the acetabulum, signifying a dislocated but reducible hip. The process is then repeated on the right hip with the left hip locked against the pelvis in abduction. The infant is positioned similarly for performance of the Barlow test; however, the thumb is positioned at the distal medial thigh and is used to apply a gentle lateral and downward force at the hip joint in an attempt to dislocate the femoral head from the acetabulum. When the hip is displaced from the acetabulum, the hip is described as dislocatable. When the Barlow test results in positioning of the femoral head within the confines of the acetabulum, the hip is described as subluxatable. After 3 months of age, the Ortolani and Barlow tests become difficult to elicit because progressive soft tissue contracture evolves and the so-called secondary signs develop the risk of restriction of abduction, leg length asymmetry, and a limp (after walking age). The secondary signs may not appear until after 9 months of age.

Radiographic Evaluation

In normal newborns with clinical evidence of DDH, routine radiography of the hips and pelvis may be confirmatory, but a normal radiograph does not exclude the presence of instability; in fact, the cartilaginous nature of the hip joint infers little value to normal radiographs. The current gold standard for imaging of the neonatal hip is ultrasonography, as described by Graf[17–19] and subsequently by Novick[30] and Clarke and Harcke.[31,32]

Ultrasonography

Diagnostic ultrasonography uses a transducer that functions as a transmitter and a receiver of acoustic energy. Ultrasonography of infant hips uses a real-time scanning technique in which ultrasonographic pulses are transmitted into the body and are received rapidly enough so that the movement of mobile anatomic structures can be observed directly. Ultrasonography offers distinct advantages compared with other imaging techniques. First, unlike plain radiography, it can distinguish the cartilaginous components of the acetabulum and the femoral head from other soft tissue structures. Second, real-time ultrasonography permits multiplanar examinations that can clearly determine the position of the femoral head with respect to the acetabulum; thus, it provides the same type of information that can be obtained with arthrography, computerized tomography, or magnetic resonance imaging but at a lower cost. Third, ultrasonography does not require sedation and does not involve ionizing radiation. Finally, unlike other techniques, it allows observation of changes in hip position with movement (**Figs. 2** and **3**).[32]

The pioneering work by Graf[17–19] emphasized a morphologic approach to the ultrasonographic examination based on a coronal image obtained through a lateral approach when the infant is in the lateral decubitus position; Novick[30] and then Harcke and colleagues[31,32] developed a technique based on a dynamic multiplanar examination that assesses the hip in positions produced by the Ortolani and Barlow maneuvers. The dynamic approach can also be used to assess acetabular morphology and development; however, it places the greatest emphasis on the position and stability of the femoral head. These two approaches are not in conflict with one another; currently, most clinicians perform what has been termed the dynamic standard minimum examination, which includes assessment in the coronal plane with the hip at rest and assessment in the transverse plane with the hip under stress. With regard to the specifics of these elements, some options are left to the preference of the examiner. It should be noted that the measurement of acetabular characteristics, such as angular measurement of acetabular landmarks, is considered optional.[32–37]

The static technique is performed with the infant in the lateral decubitus position and the hip in 35° of flexion and 10° of internal rotation.[37] Morphology is assessed by describing basic anatomic features and by angular measurement. The dynamic hip examination is performed following an examination of the hip at rest. The hip is checked for instability, which can be quantified by measurement of the degree of displacement of the femoral head. The infant lies on his or her side in the positioning apparatus and the transducer is positioned over the hip, which is then adducted and pushed superiorly to demonstrate

instability. Angular measurements serve to confirm the diagnosis indicated by the morphologic description and provide a quantitative parameter for comparison of findings (**Fig. 4**).[17,30,31,37]

A coronal image of the hip is obtained and 3 lines are constructed: a vertical line drawn parallel to the ossified lateral wall of the ilium, termed the base line; a line drawn from the inferior edge of the osseous acetabulum (the inferior iliac margin) at the roof of the triradiate cartilage to the most lateral point on the ilium (the superior osseous rim), termed the bony roofline; and a line drawn along the roof of the cartilaginous acetabulum, from the lateral osseous edge of the acetabulum to the labrum, termed the cartilage roofline. Two angles are calculated. The α angle is formed by the intersection of the base line and the bony roofline. The lower limit of normal for the α angle is 60°. This angle reflects osseous coverage of the femoral head by the acetabulum; the smaller the angle the greater the degree of dysplasia. The β angle is formed by the intersection of the base line and the cartilage roofline. The upper limit of normal for the β angle is 55°. The β angle reflects cartilaginous coverage of the femoral head; the greater the angle the greater the degree of dislocation.[17]

Graf[17–19] has classified hips according to the measurements based on the degree of femoral head displacement and the associated deformation and growth retardation of the acetabular roof. Type I indicates a normal hip with a good cartilaginous and osseous roof (an α angle of 60° or more). Type IIa represents an immature hip in an infant who is younger than 3 months with delayed ossification but an adequate cartilaginous roof and an α angle of 50° to 59°. Type IIb refers to a hip with delayed ossification in an infant older than 3 months with a rounded osseous acetabular promontory; an α angle of 50° to 59° and a β angle

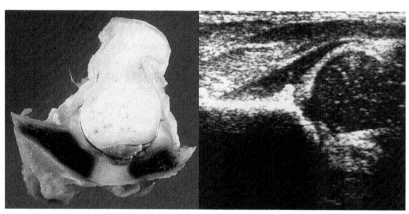

Fig. 2. Ultrasound scan in standard plane with anatomic section for comparison.

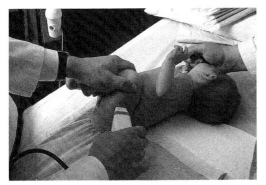

Fig. 3. Dynamic ultrasound scan technique with stress maneuver in process.

of more than 55°. Types IIc, III, and IV are always pathologic. In types III and IV, the bone molding of the acetabulum is severely deficient or poor and there is lateralization of the femoral head. The α angle is 43° to 49° in type IIc and less than 43° in types III and IV. The β angle is 70° to 77° in type IIc and more than 77° in type III and IV. Angular measurement is subject to interobserver and intraobserver error. In type IV, the cartilaginous acetabulum is interposed between the femoral head and the ilium. Regardless of the hip type, testing for instability should always be performed.[37]

The technique of dynamic hip ultrasonography incorporates motion and stress maneuvers that are based on accepted clinical examination techniques (**Fig. 5**). With the dynamic method, an attempt is made to visualize the Barlow and Ortolani maneuvers on the ultrasonography screen.

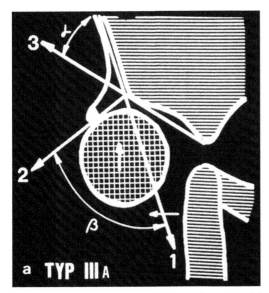

Fig. 4. Graf type III. An ultrasound scan with measurements.

The technique depends on ligamentous or capsular laxity; as with the physical examination, the study quality depends on the operator performing the stress test. In a normal hip, the femoral head is well positioned and stable under stress. In the first few weeks of life, the femoral head is reduced in the acetabulum at rest but it may show slight displacement (physiologic laxity) under stress; this should resolve by the time the infant is 4 weeks of age. Although subluxation implies displacement of the head from the acetabulum, the head is not completely dislocated. In more severe forms of hip dysplasia, the femoral head may be dislocated from the acetabulum at rest (but may be reduced with maneuvers) or it may be displaced by means of maneuvers. An image is obtained with the hip flexed to 90° as posterior stress is applied to the knee with the palm of the hand the Barlow provocative test (see **Fig. 3**); any resultant subluxation is then noted (see **Figs. 4** and **5**). It should be remembered that 4 to 6 mm of subluxation is normal during the first few days of life.[38] If the hip subluxates or dislocates, reduction is attempted (the Ortolani maneuver).[33–36]

The morphologic technique provides information related to the development of the femoral head and the acetabulum. Development of the ossification center of the femoral head is an important landmark recognized between 2 and 8 months of age. The ages at which the ossification center normally appears range widely and it typically develops earlier in girls. The femoral ossification center is detected on the ultrasonogram before it is visible radiographically. With maturation, the ossification center increases in size until it becomes large enough to obscure the echoes from the inferior iliac margin at the medial part of the acetabulum. Because of the maturation process, the real-time scan is not capable of demonstrating details of the key anatomic landmarks and, with increasing age, it loses its advantage compared with plain radiography for the recognition of anatomic structures.

TREATMENT

Debate continues concerning which clinically and sonographically abnormal hips require intervention and by what age.

- Many hips have some degree of instability at birth, demonstrable on ultrasound, which often corrects spontaneously and may be observed for 3 weeks without treatment. Observation is permissible for instability and subluxation up to 6 weeks and for sonographic acetabular growth retardation.

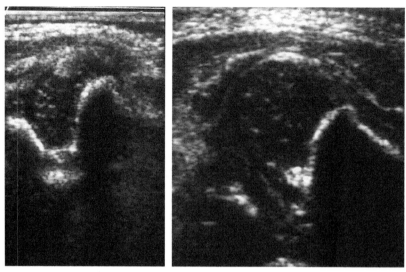

Fig. 5. Dynamic ultrasound transverse flexion view with stress on the right side.

- The triple-diaper technique, which prevents hip adduction, is still used but has demonstrated no improvement in results compared with no intervention at all in the first 3 weeks of life.
- Treatment is indicated when evidence of subluxation of the hip persists beyond 3 weeks on physical examination or ultrasonographic evaluation.
- When actual hip dislocation is noted at birth, treatment is indicated without need for an observation period.[36–38]
- Treatment is indicated in hips that are clinically stable but at 6 weeks still have an abnormal ultrasound. Criteria for treatment on the ultrasound may differ from center to center. The authors consider treatment at 6 weeks if the acetabulum seems morphologically immature, there is any instability detected on ultrasound, or an alpha angle is less than or equal to 57°.
- Various devices have been used for the treatment of hip instability in infants, including hip spica casts, the Frejka pillow, the Craig splint, the Ilfeld splint, and the Von Rosen splint; however, the most commonly used device by far is the Pavlik harness.

The harness is a dynamic positioning device that allows the child to move freely within the confines of its restraints. It consists of a circumferential chest strap with shoulder straps that provide sites of attachment for lower-extremity straps. The function of the anterior lower-extremity straps is to flex the hips, whereas the posterior lower-extremity straps prevent adduction of the hips. The posterior lower-extremity straps should not be used to produce abduction of the hips, which is associated with avascular necrosis. The harness should be placed with the hips in 90° to 100° of flexion and unforced spontaneous abduction with neutral or 15° of external rotation during the reduction phase and should be maintained in 90° of flexion and 45° of abduction in the maintenance phase. Indications for the use of the Pavlik harness include the presence of a reducible hip in an infant who is not yet making attempts to sit. The child's family must be able to follow instructions and be available for frequent evaluations and harness adjustments. Patients must be followed up closely at weekly (or at least every 2 weeks) intervals to avoid complications. If the hip is not reduced in 2 weeks by this technique, other methods of treatment should be pursued. A general rule of thumb for time in treatment when the hip is successfully reduced is the child's age at hip stability plus 3 months (**Fig. 6**).[39–41] In summary

- The harness is used for hip instability preferably between 2 to 6 weeks and up to 3 months of age.
- Initially, it should be used full time; then a weaning program is commenced only after the hip has been reduced for a minimum of 6 weeks.
- Careful follow-up is mandatory with ultrasound monitoring.

Problems with the use of the Pavlik harness can generally be attributed to compliance issues, either from parental misunderstanding or physician misuse. Complications directly related to use of the harness are rare but can include transient femoral neuropathy caused by persistent

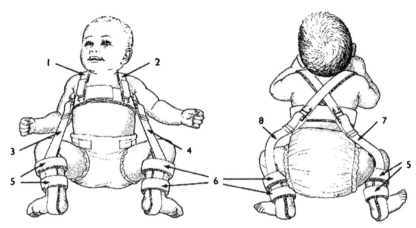

Fig. 6. Pavlik harness: drawing from a parental instruction manual. (*Courtesy of* Southampton General Hospital, Southampton, UK.)

hyperflexion of the hips and avascular necrosis caused by excessive abduction, which should be avoided; avascular necrosis is rare, with a reported incidence of less than 1%.[42] Another problem related to misuse of the harness occurs when a hip is not adequately reduced and rests on the posterior lip of the acetabulum for a prolonged period, this can cause blunting of the acetabulum and a form of dysplasia (termed Pavlik harness disease), which is difficult to treat. These complications are rare and can be avoided with close follow-up and parental involvement.[41]

Finally, there is a significant range in treatment rates depending on ultrasound technique and geographic location. In Germany, the treatment rate is 60 per 1000. Clarke and colleagues[43] have reported a rate of 7.2 per 1000 after ultrasound screening for infants at risk, with a surgical treatment rate of 0.74 per 1000.

Closed reduction with examination of the hips under general anesthesia is reserved for those children in whom concentric reduction cannot be achieved with simpler methods. If stable concentric reduction of the hip joint is not attained after a trial period of 2 weeks in the Pavlik harness, this method should be abandoned. Closed reduction and hip spica casting may also be the treatment of choice for patients with an unreliable family or unfavorable social situation. Fixed abduction braces are commonly used in Europe for residual dysplasia after hip repositioning in the harness.[44–46]

SUMMARY

Early diagnosis is of paramount importance to favorably alter the natural history of DDH. Most cases of dysplasia can be diagnosed by careful history taking and physical examination. Imaging modalities, such as ultrasonography,

have increased our ability to detect subtleties not appreciated by means of physical examination or plain radiography.

Although the evaluation of children with risk factors for DDH is important, most dysplasia occurs in girls who have no other risk factors. For all infants, a competent newborn physical examination using the Ortolani maneuver is the most useful procedure to detect hip instability. Early treatment of an unstable hip with a Pavlik harness or similarly effective orthosis is effective, safe, and strongly advised.

FUTURE PERSPECTIVE

Our knowledge of DDH continues to evolve. With advanced screening strategies, most cases can be detected early and optimal treatment decided by 6 weeks. In the future, most national health systems should implement clinical guidelines for the early detection and treatment of dysplasia because untreated dysplasia continues to be a significant burden on the cost of health. Improvements in the technology related to ultrasonography and further training will allow improved imaging and reduce the complication rate. The incidence of dysplasia will not be reduced in the foreseeable future; however, advancements in detection should make dysplasia a condition that is easily treatable and practically no cases should go undetected or untreated.

In summary, the most important strategies are to improve nonoperative childhood management and these are

- Early diagnosis before 6 weeks
- Early supervised treatment with ultrasound monitoring
- The coordinated approach and dedicated staff

- Familiarity with the spectrum of pathologic conditions of developmental dysplasia, both clinically and sonographically
- Competence in ultrasound technique and interpretation

REFERENCES

1. Kocher MS. Ultrasonographic screening for developmental dysplasia of the hip: an epidemiologic analysis (part I). Am J Orthop 2000;29:929–33.
2. Andren L, Borglin NE. A disorder of oestrogen metabolism as a causal factor of congenital dislocation of the hip. Acta Orthop Scand 1960;30:169–71.
3. Aronsson DD, Goldberg MJ, Kling TF Jr, et al. Developmental dysplasia of the hip. Pediatrics 1994; 94(2 pt 1):201–8.
4. Dunn PM. Perinatal observations on the etiology of congenital dislocation of the hip. Clin Orthop 1976; 119:11–22.
5. Klisic PJ. Congenital dislocation of the hip: a misleading term – brief report. J Bone Joint Surg Br 1989;71:136.
6. Barlow TG. Early diagnosis and treatment of congenital dislocation of the hip. J Bone Joint Surg Br 1962;44:292–301.
7. Vitale MG, Skaggs DL. Developmental dysplasia of the hip from six months to four years of age. J Am Acad Orthop Surg 2001;9(6):401–41.
8. Sankar WN, Weiss J, Skaggs DL. Orthopaedic conditions in the newborn. J Am Acad Orthop Surg 2009;17(2):112–22.
9. Guille JT, Pizzutillo PD, MacEwen GD. Developmental dysplasia of the hip from birth to six months. J Am Acad Orthop Surg 2000;8:232–42.
10. Rosendahl K, Markestad T, Lie RT. Ultrasound in the early diagnosis of congenital dislocation of the hip: the significance of hip stability versus acetabular morphology. Pediatr Radiol 1992;22:430–3.
11. Patel H. Canadian Task Force on Preventive Health Care. Preventive health care, 2001 update: screening and management of developmental dysplasia of the hip in newborns. CMAJ 2001;164:1669–77.
12. Shipman SA, Helfand M, Moyer VA, et al. Screening for developmental dysplasia of the hip: a systematic literature review for the US Preventive Services Task Force. Pediatrics 2006;117:E557–76.
13. Gage JR, Winter RB. Avascular necrosis of the capital femoral epiphysis as a complication of closed reduction of congenital dislocation of the hip. A critical review of twenty years' experience at Gillette Children's Hospital. J Bone Joint Surg Am 1972;54:373–88.
14. Yoshitaka T, Mitani S, Aoki K, et al. Long-term follow-up of congenital subluxation of the hip. J Pediatr Orthop 2001;21:474–80.
15. Harris WH. Etiology of osteoarthritis of the hip. Clin Orthop Relat Res 1986;213:20–33.
16. Felson DT, Zhang Y. An update on the epidemiology of knee and hip osteoarthritis with a view to prevention. Arthritis Rheum 1998;41:1343–55.
17. Graf R. The diagnosis of congenital hip-joint dislocation by the ultrasonic compound treatment. Arch Orthop Trauma Surg 1980;97:117–33.
18. Graf R. Fundamentals of sonographic diagnosis of infant hip dysplasia. J Pediatr Orthop 1984;4: 735–40.
19. Graf R. New possibilities for the diagnosis of congenital hip joint dislocation by ultrasonography. J Pediatr Orthop 1983;3:354–9.
20. Rosendahl K, Markestad T, Lie RT. Ultrasound screening for developmental dysplasia of the hip in the neonate: the effect on treatment rate and prevalence of late cases. Pediatrics 1994;94: 47–52.
21. Clinical practice guideline: early detection of developmental dysplasia of the hip. Committee on Quality Improvement, Subcommittee on Developmental Dysplasia of the Hip. American Academy of Pediatrics. Pediatrics 2000;105(4 Pt 1):896–905.
22. Lehmann HP, Hinton R, Morello P, et al. Developmental dysplasia of the hip practice guideline: technical report. Committee on Quality Improvement, and Subcommittee on Developmental Dysplasia of the Hip. Pediatrics 2000;105:E57.
23. Goldberg M. Early detection of developmental hip dysplasia: synopsis of the AAP clinical practice guideline. Pediatr Rev 2001;22:131–4.
24. US Preventive Services Task Force. Screening for developmental dysplasia of the hip: recommendation statement. Pediatrics 2006;117:898–902.
25. Mahan ST, Katz JN, Kim YJ. To screen or not to screen? A decision analysis of the utility of screening for developmental dysplasia of the hip. J Bone Joint Surg Am 2009;91:1705–19.
26. Schwend RM, Schoenecker P, Richards BS, et al. Screening the newborn for developmental dysplasia of the hip: now what do we do? J Pediatr Orthop 2007;27(6):607–10.
27. Hummer CD Jr, MacEwen GD. The coexistence of torticollis and congenital dysplasia of the hip. J Bone Joint Surg Am 1972;54:1255–6.
28. Kumar SJ, MacEwen GD. The incidence of hip dysplasia with metatarsus adductus. Clin Orthop 1982;164:234–5.
29. Bond CD, Hennrikus WL, DellaMaggiore ED. Prospective evaluation of newborn soft-tissue hip 'clicks' with ultrasound. J Pediatr Orthop 1997;17:199–201.
30. Novick G, Ghelman B, Schneider M. Sonography of the neonatal and infant hip. Am J Roentgenol 1983; 141:639–45.
31. Clarke NM, Harcke HT, McHugh P, et al. Real time ultrasound in the diagnosis of congenital dislocation

and dysplasia of the hip. J Bone Joint Surg Br 1985; 67(3):406–12.

32. Harcke HT, Kumar SJ. The role of ultrasound in the diagnosis and management of congenital dislocation and dysplasia of the hip. J Bone Joint Surg Am 1991;73:622–8.

33. Donaldson JS, Feinstein KA. Imaging of developmental dysplasia of the hip. Pediatr Clin North Am 1997;44:591–614.

34. Harcke HT, Graf R, Clarke NM. Program and abstracts of the consensus meeting on hip sonography. Wilmington (DE): Alfred I. duPont Institute; 1993. p. 23–4.

35. Harcke HT, Grissom LE. Infant hip sonography: current concepts. Semin Ultrasound CT MR 1994; 15:256–63.

36. Harcke HT. Ultrasound of the pediatric hip. In: Taveras JM, Ferrucci JT, editors. Radiology, diagnosis - imaging - intervention. New York: Lippincott-Raven; 1997.

37. Wientroub S, Grill F. Ultrasonography in developmental dysplasia of the hip. J Bone Joint Surg Am 2000;82:1004–18.

38. Devred P, Tréguier C, Ducou-Le-Pointe H. Echography of the hip and other imaging techniques in pediatrics. J Radiol 2001;82:803–16.

39. Ramsey PL, Lasser S, MacEwen GD. Congenital dislocation of the hip: use of the Pavlik harness in the child during the first six months of life. J Bone Joint Surg Am 1976;58:1000–4.

40. Kalamchi A, MacFarlane R III. The Pavlik harness: results in patients over three months of age. J Pediatr Orthop 1982;2:3–8.

41. Mubarak S, Garfin S, Vance R, et al. Pitfalls in the use of the Pavlik harness for treatment of congenital dysplasia, subluxation, and dislocation of the hip. J Bone Joint Surg Am 1981;63:1239–48.

42. Clarke NM, Reading IC, Corbin C, et al. Twenty years' experience of selective secondary ultrasound screening for congenital dislocation of the hip. Arch Dis Child 2012;97:423–9.

43. Harris IE, Dickens R, Menelaus MB. Use of the Pavlik harness for hip displacements. When to abandon treatment. Clin Orthop Relat Res 1992;281:29–33.

44. Ishii Y, Ponseti IV. Long-term results of closed reduction of complete congenital dislocation of the hip in children under one year of age. Clin Orthop 1978; 137:167–74.

45. Malvitz TA, Weinstein SL. Closed reduction for congenital dysplasia of the hip: functional and radiographic results after an average of thirty years. J Bone Joint Surg Am 1994;76:1777–92.

46. Luhmann SJ, Schoenecker PL, Anderson AM, et al. The prognostic importance of the ossific nucleus in the treatment of congenital dysplasia of the hip. J Bone Joint Surg Am 1998;80:1719–27.

Strategies to Improve Outcomes from Operative Childhood Management of DDH

John H. Wedge, O.C., MD, FRCSC*,
Simon P. Kelley, MBChB, FRCS (Tr and Orth)

KEYWORDS

• DDH • Open reduction • Redislocation • Avascular necrosis

KEY POINTS

- Outcomes from the operative management of developmental dysplasia of the hip (DDH) are highly dependent on 2 major factors: first, the ability of a surgeon to accurately assess DDH and select the appropriate surgical procedure, and, second, the skill and precision with which the surgery is performed.
- Postoperative redislocation after open reduction is in most cases a preventable complication that can be avoided by adhering to surgical principles outlined in this article.
- The next most important complication or sequela in the surgical management of DDH is avascular necrosis (AVN). This is an iatrogenic problem because it is not seen in the natural history of DDH.

INTRODUCTION

Outcomes from the operative management of DDH are highly dependent on 2 major factors: first, the ability of a surgeon to accurately assess DDH and select the appropriate surgical procedure and, second, the skill and precision with which the surgery is performed. AVN or osteonecrosis and growth disturbance may result from intrinsic or extrinsic factors and are often unavoidable iatrogenic sequela of open or closed hip reduction. Redislocations may be unavoidable but surgical technique is nevertheless important.

Postoperative redislocation after open reduction is in most cases a preventable complication that can be avoided by adhering to surgical principles outlined in this article. Redislocation has the potential to compromise all future attempts at restoring normal function to the hip. The first section of this article addresses how to avoid this devastating complication by highlighting some key steps in the surgical technique of open reduction of the dislocated hip. The second section discusses how to decide when to add a pelvic osteotomy, a femoral osteotomy, or both to enhance the stability of the newly reduced hip. The third section of this article outlines how to salvage the hip that has suffered a redislocation.

The next most important complication or sequela in the surgical management of DDH is AVN. This is an iatrogenic problem because it is not seen in the natural history of DDH. The fourth section of this article discusses strategies to reduce the AVN rate and, finally, the fifth section describes how to manage it when it does occur.

PREVENTING REDISLOCATION OF THE HIP AFTER OPEN REDUCTION THROUGH AN ANTERIOR APPROACH

The following are the major reasons why a hip may redislocate postoperatively:

1. Failure to identify and expose the true acetabulum and achieve a concentric reduction.

Division of Orthopaedic Surgery, The Hospital for Sick Children, 555 University Ave, Toronto M5GIX8, Canada
* Corresponding author.
E-mail address: john.wedge@sickkids.ca

Orthop Clin N Am 43 (2012) 291–299
doi:10.1016/j.ocl.2012.05.003
0030-5898/12/$ – see front matter © 2012 Elsevier Inc. All rights reserved.

A thorough knowledge of the pathoanatomy of a child's dislocated hip is crucial to successfully achieving adequate exposure of the true acetabulum and achieving a concentric reduction. The authors have found it helpful to use a surgical headlamp to assist with visualization during open reductions. Using a standard Smith-Peterson approach through a bikini line incision, the anterior aspect of the hip must be exposed to the medial aspect of the acetabulum and laterally to the level of the apex of the dislocated femoral head. After dividing the long head of rectus femoris just distal to its attachment to the anterior inferior iliac spine, the surgeon should spend time fully exposing the anterior aspect of the hip joint capsule. Unless excellent exposure of the hip joint capsule is achieved one cannot hope to perform a well-placed capsulotomy to visualize the true acetabulum. The exposure involves 2 key maneuvers. The first is to develop a plane of dissection superolaterally between the joint capsule and the hip abductors along the line of the reflected head of rectus femoris. This tissue plane can then be connected to the subperiosteal plane previously developed along the lateral aspect of the ilium using curved Mayo scissors. The second maneuver is to develop the tissue plane across the anterior aspect of the hip joint capsule. The iliopsoas tendon is firmly adherent to the anterior capsule at this point and it is critical to bluntly dissect this plane, such that a Langenbeck retractor or Hohmann retractor may be placed medial to the true acetabulum between the iliopsoas tendon and the anterior capsule. The authors find that the combination of a spade-shaped periosteal elevator and a large swab are ideal instruments to achieve this step in a safe and controlled manner. Failure to free the iliopsoas from the capsule at this point compromises the ability to extend the medial aspect of the capsulotomy to expose the true acetabulum despite performing an iliopsoas tenotomy over the pelvic brim. The iliopsoas tendon is recessed just proximal to the musculotendinous junction. The surgeon should avoid transection of the femoral nerve, which lies just medial and anterior to the tendon. Great care is required to ensure an accurate capsulotomy, which should follow the line of the acetabulum, approximately 5 mm to 8 mm distal to its edge. A common error is to veer too inferiorly with the medial aspect of the capsulotomy, thus leaving a tight band of capsular tissue anteriorly, preventing clear visualization of the true acetabulum and even preventing concentric reduction of the femoral head. This can be avoided by using a Macdonald elevator to probe the anteromedial aspect of the acetabulum through the initial small anterior capsulotomy to guide the surgeon as to the correct medial extension of the capsulotomy. After opening the capsule, the ligamentum teres should be identified from its origin on the femoral head and traced down to its insertion at the fovea of the true acetabulum, which should now be clearly seen under direct vision. If it is not clearly seen, there is usually inadequate medial dissection and capsullotomy. The adjacent medial capsule and transverse acetabular ligament must be cut because these structures are always contracted in a hip that has been dislocated for a significant length of time.

2. Excessive tension across the hip joint.

Adductor tenotomy and iliopsoas recession are integral steps to relieve tension across the joint. The actual reduction of the femoral head into the acetabulum should not be a forceful event. In most children over the age of 30 months, a femoral shortening osteotomy is necessary to bring the femoral head to the level of the acetabulum. It is important to remove sufficient bone (typically 1–2 cm) such that the femoral head may be reduced without too much tension. Doing so also reduces the likelihood of AVN. It is better, however, to err on the side of initially resecting too little bone and subsequently adjusting the tension by removing a little more as necessary.

3. Inadequate tension across the hip joint to maintain stability.

There is a tendency to remove too long a segment of bone from the femur, thereby compromising the postoperative stability of the hip. It is often recommended to reduce the femoral head after the femoral osteotomy and then to remove the amount of bone that is overlapping. This maneuver often suggests resecting a larger segment of bone than is actually necessary. To avoid this catastrophic occurrence, moderate traction should be applied to the leg before determining the amount to be resected. It is rare that more than 2 cm of bone needs to be resected.

4. Abnormal version of the proximal femur.

A marked increase in femoral anteversion is not universal in DDH after walking age. Bilateral, high, posterior dislocations may be associated with femoral retroversion. First, the associated abnormality of version must be assessed intraoperatively in each child, and, second, great care must be taken with the amount of correction (derotation) placed at the osteotomy site. The most common technical error is overcorrection, leaving the proximal femur retroverted, leading to posterior subluxation or dislocation postoperatively. A helpful rule is to never correct the anteversion to less than 20°. Dividing the estimated amount of anteversion present in half and then externally rotating the leg at the osteotomy by this amount best achieves this goal. The explanation for this is because of the windlass effect on the soft tissues with femoral rotation. After significant rotational realignment, the total arc of rotation at the hip is reduced by the increase in soft tissue tension generated. Failure to recognize and correct excessive femoral anteversion may lead to gradual subluxation of the hip after cast removal. The leg is typically internally rotated in the cast and when postimmobilization stiffness resolves and the leg externally rotates back to neutral, the hip may subluxate anteriorly.

5. Failure to redirect the acetabulum into the proper position.

Inadequate correction of the acetabular dysplasia with an acetabuloplasty or a Salter innominate osteotomy may cause persistent instability and resubluxation in the cast. Overcorrection (more likely with a triple innominate osteotomy) may leave posterior acetabular wall deficiency and posterior dislocation that may not be recognized intraoperatively.

6. Tying the sutures in the capsular repair before fixation of the femoral and/or pelvic osteotomies.

If performing a one-stage open reduction and osteotomy, tying the capsular repair should always be the last step of the operation, before wound closure, to ensure a secure reduction. Pelvic and femoral osteotomies result in an alteration of the morphology of the hip joint. A capsulorrhaphy performed before these osteotomies loses tension, leading to immediate loss of stability, and may subsequently lead to redislocation.

7. Loss of control of the operated hip in the transition from end of the surgical procedure to the application of the hip spica cast.

The operating surgeon should be in complete control of the newly reduced hip at all times. This is particularly important when the superficial tissue layers are being closed and preparations are made to apply a hip spica cast. There can be a loss of concentration of the surgical team combined with the child being repositioned that may lead to an unidentified perioperative redislocation. The operating surgeon must maintain control of the leg throughout this period of transition to ensure reduction is held and to identify redislocation while coordinating the rest of the team to prepare the spica cast.

8. Inadequate molding of the spica cast over the greater trochanter.

The hip spica cast is an important element of the comprehensive operative management of the dislocated hip. A spica cast can maintain reduction of a more unstable hip if expertly applied by the use of molding to support the hip. Using the thenar eminence, the cast should be molded carefully over the lateral and posterior aspect of the greater trochanter to ensure there is no dead space (as indicated by a gap between soft tissue and cast on postoperative imaging) that compromises the stability of the hip.

Dislocations in children with a poorly defined margin between the true acetabulum and false acetabulum and a high acetabular index may be difficult to completely stabilize using a standard menu of open reduction, capsulorrhaphy, and osteotomies (**Fig. 1**A). If there is still a tendency of the femoral head to slide proximally after fixation of the osteotomy(ies) and repair of the capsule even with the leg in a position of maximal stability, then it is occasionally necessary to use extra-articular fixation from the greater trochanter to the ilium proximal to the pelvic osteotomy. This is achieved using a large threaded Steinmann pin or Kirschner wire, which can be removed through a window in the spica cast at 4 to 6 weeks postoperatively (see **Fig. 1**E).

WHEN SHOULD A PELVIC OR FEMORAL OSTEOTOMY BE DONE WITH AN OPEN REDUCTION FOR DDH?

An important decision in the management of DDH is whether to add a femoral or pelvic osteotomy or both to an open reduction in a child after walking age. In the authors' opinion, a pelvic osteotomy is almost always necessary in a child of walking age to avoid future surgery for residual dysplasia that may be as a high as 80%[1] when a pelvic osteotomy is not done as an integral part of the primary procedure. A second and perhaps more compelling reason for a concomitant pelvic osteotomy is to enhance the stability of the open reduction. Careful intraoperative assessment of the location, extent, and direction of the acetabular orientation and deficiency informs the decision as to the type of pelvic osteotomy required. If a deficiency is principally anterolateral and the hypoplastic true acetabulum has a uniform radius, then a redirectional acetabular osteotomy, such as the Salter innominate osteotomy, is indicated. If there is a more lateral deficiency, however, where the dislocating femoral head has exited the true acetabulum, there is erosion of the margin of the

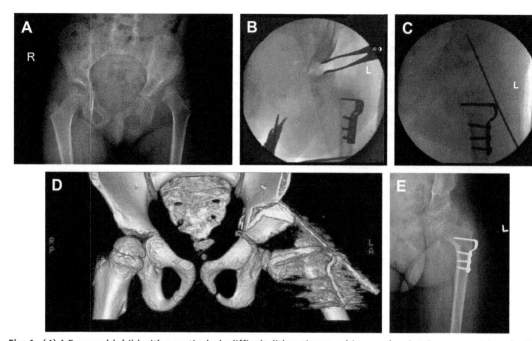

Fig. 1. (A) A 5-year-old child with a particularly difficult dislocation to achieve and maintain a concentric reduction. The lateral margin of the true acetabulum has been eroded making it almost continuous with the false acetabulum. The medial aspect of the femoral head is flattened further complicating achieving concentricity after reduction. (B) Intraoperative image after a varus derotation osteotomy of the femur and a periacetabular osteotomy before insertion of a bone graft obtained form the femoral osteotomy site. (C) After a capsulorrhaphy, the hip was not completely stable due to the very hypoplastic acetabulum. Therefore, a smooth Kirschner wire was passed subcutaneously through the greater trochanter into the ilium proximal to the osteotomy to stabilize the hip. This was removed through a window in the cast 4 weeks postoperatively. Intra-articular pins should be avoided because of damage to the articular cartilage and the risk of septic arthritis. (D) Postoperative CT scan demonstrating Toronto version of a periacetabular osteotomy and concentric reduction of the hip. (E) Two years later, she had a normal gait, excellent range of motion, and equal leg lengths. Note the Harris, or growth arrest, line in the proximal femoral metaphysis indicating lack of growth disturbance. There is no evidence of osteonecrosis of the epiphysis.

true acetabulum, and if there is a steeply sloping and flat medial wall, then an acetabular volume-altering osteotomy, such as the Dega osteotomy or Pemberton osteotomy, is preferred. After completion of the pelvic osteotomy and reduction of the femoral head, before tying the sutures placed for the capsulorrhaphy, improved stability of the hip in only slight flexion, internal rotation, and minimal abduction should be evident. If not, then postoperative problems with stability of the hip should be anticipated.

As discussed previously, a derotation osteotomy of the femur may need to be added in a 1-year-old to 3-year-old child if there is marked femoral anteversion (>50°) to also enhance postoperative stability of the hip. This can be identified either at the commencement of the surgery, by performing an examination of the proximal femur under fluoroscopic control or under direct examination of the proximal femur after capsulotomy. After 30 months of age, a femoral shortening osteotomy is almost always required to facilitate the open reduction, prevent excessive pressure on the femoral head

causing AVN, correct excessive femoral anteversion, and improve the intraoperative stability of the hip.

SALVAGE OF THE REDISLOCATED HIP AFTER OPEN REDUCTION

If a postoperative CT or MRI scan reveals resubluxation or dislocation, re-exploration of the hip and revision of the open reduction and osteotomy(ies) should be done on an urgent basis. It should not be delayed with the futile hope that the hip will spontaneously stabilize. The likelihood of successful salvage diminishes considerably after several weeks. The surgeon needs to identify the cause of the redislocation and aim to correct it accordingly. The cause is likely to be either that the hip was never completely exposed and reduced during the index surgery or one of the factors identified previously in this article.

If redislocation is identified after cast removal, typically at 2 to 3 months post–open reduction, then a different approach is necessary. At this stage, the hip is typically stiff, the skin is in poor health, and the bone around the hip very osteopenic. Operating at this stage is not recommended. It is best to allow the hip to mobilize and regain range of motion and to allow the bone density time to recover with return to normal activity by the child. This typically takes to 2 to 3 months. In the meantime, planning for repeat open reduction includes a CT scan of the hip with 3-D reconstructions and a femoral anteversion study to assess the location of the femoral head, the possible presence of proximal femoral valgus deformity, the orientation of the acetabulum, and potential displacement or incorrect original alignment of the pelvic osteotomy. Careful assessment of femoral version is essential because one of the most common problems is posterior dislocation of the femoral head due to excessive derotation of the femur at the original procedure.

Salvage of a redislocation is one of the most technically demanding of procedures in pediatric hip surgery because of distorted anatomy, dense fibrous scar tissue close to vital structures (nerves and blood vessels), and poor bone quality. **Fig. 2** illustrates a redislocation referred more than 8 months after the index procedure. The surgeon had treated the child in an abduction brace for months after recognizing the redislocation with

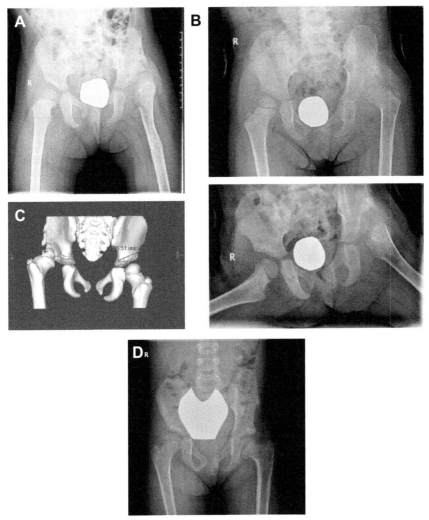

Fig. 2. (A) This child presented at age 3, 8 months after open reduction and osteotomies. The surgeon had removed metal but failed to relocate the hip. (B) Radiographs immediately before revision surgery. Because her hip had been continuously immobilized since her original surgery with marked osteoporosis and stiffness, the authors waited 3 months for her bone to strengthen and regain mobility of the hip joint. (C) Preoperative CT scan demonstrating osteonecrosis of the proximal femoral epiphysis and the femoral head situated in a false osteotomy. (D) Four years postrevision of the open reduction and femoral and pelvic osteotomies. Range of motion is full except she has only 25° of internal rotation, equal leg lengths, and normal gait.

the hope that the hip would spontaneously improve. Of particular importance when reoperating is to carefully avoid damaging the lateral acetabular epiphysis while locating the true acetabulum. This structure, which is critical to normal acetabular development in adolescence, is often damaged in re-exploration procedures.

PREVENTION OF AVASCULAR NECROSIS AND GROWTH DISTURBANCE

AVN is an iatrogenic complication or sequela of the treatment of DDH that even in its mildest form compromises the longevity of the hip[2] in adulthood. It may be as frequent as 43% after open reduction.[3] Fortunately, AVN is compatible with satisfactory function until the late teenage or adult years and many hips function well despite the defrmity.[4] It is not likely to be possible to completely eliminate AVN as a complication of the operative management of a DDH but adhering to the surgical principles described in this article can reduce the incidence.[5]

Adductor tenotomy, iliopsoas recession, extensive medial capsular release, division of the transverse acetabular ligament, and femoral shortening osteotomy during an open reduction of a dislocated hip through an anterior approach may reduce tension across the hip joint and compressive forces on the soft femoral head of early childhood. Medial approaches to the hip joint have the potential for a higher rate of AVN because the medial femoral circumflex artery and its lateral epiphyseal branches are inevitably damaged to some degree by the exposure even if only by retraction during the operation. The medial femoral circumflex artery is the main blood supply to the proximal femoral epiphysis in the age group of children typically presenting with a dislocated hip. Surgeons should not rely on extreme positioning within a spica cast, in particular abduction of more than 30°, to provide postoperative stability to the hip joint after open reduction, because this may compromise the circulation to the femoral head and lead to AVN.

MANAGEMENT OF THE SEQUELAE OF AVASCULAR NECROSIS AFTER OPEN REDUCTION
Early

AVN may have a deleterious effect on hip development throughout growth, leading to incongruity of the joint and arthritis early in adult life.[6] Even milder forms (Kalamchi and MacEwen or Bucholz and

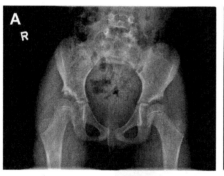
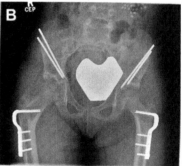
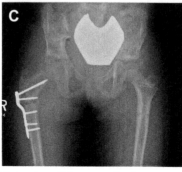

Fig. 3. (*A*) A 4-year-old girl who had bilateral medial open reductions at 6 months of age complicated by bilateral AVN, type I on the left and type II on the right. There is persistent acetabular dysplasia more marked on the right side with subluxation of the hip. (*B*) Three years post–bilateral femoral and innominate osteotomies, the valgus of the right proximal femur has recurred due to the ongoing effect of growth disturbance of the physis. (*C*) Several weeks after repeat osteotomy of the right femur. A further osteotomy may be required later in childhood or adolescence to ensure continued acetabular development.

Ogden types I and II)[7,8] may eventually result in delayed or arrested acetabular development after open reduction despite seemingly favorable early postoperative development supported by acetabular indices within the normal range. Type II AVN with lateral arrest of the proximal femoral physis may be particularly pernicious with valgus deformity causing eccentric loading of the hip and impairment of acetabular development as early as 5 to 7 years of age (**Fig. 3**). The dysplasia may become permanent if the valgus deformity is not corrected before the appearance of the lateral acetabular epiphysis in early adolescence.

If AVN occurs after an open reduction of a dislocated hip where a concomitant pelvic osteotomy was not performed, the ensuing acetabular dysplasia is less likely to correct spontaneously. The more likely scenario is that of relentless progression of acetabular dysplasia, which only becomes more difficult to salvage in the future. In this situation, the surgeon needs to be much more aggressive to optimize the development of the acetabulum, and a pelvic osteotomy should be performed. Early correction of the dysplasia with a pelvic osteotomy also has the additional benefit of containing the damaged and biologically soft preosseous cartilage of the proximal femoral epiphysis and mitigating the deformity anticipated from the necrosis, thereby producing a more spherical femoral head (**Fig. 4**). The type of pelvic osteotomy should be chosen based on the philosophy of the treating surgeon and the morphology of the acetabular dysplasia. The Salter innominate osteotomy is ideal for anterolateral dysplasia in a congruent hip and a volume-altering acetabuloplasty more appropriate for those hips with more steep superolateral deficiency.

Late

Severe type II and types III and IV AVN may lead to pain and disability in adolescence (**Fig. 5**). Coxa breva with a deformed femoral head, short femoral neck, and overgrown greater trochanter may cause significant pain, which may be generated by intra-articular derangement, trochanteric impingement, or abductor insufficiency. Functional disability may also be caused by joint stiffness, a Trendelenburg gait, and a short leg. Complex femoral and pelvic osteotomies, often

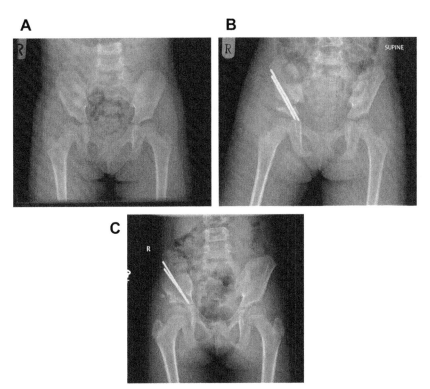

Fig. 4. (*A*) A 5-year-old girl with mild growth disturbance and failure of normal acetabular development after medial open reduction of the right hip at 4 months of age. (*B*) A right innominate osteotomy has been done to contain the vulnerable femoral head and correct the acetabular dysplasia. (*C*) At 9 years of age, the femoral head is large due to the AVN but is well contained within the acetabulum. Note the lateral acetabular epiphysis that seems to be growing well. The left hip may eventually require a pelvic osteotomy as well.

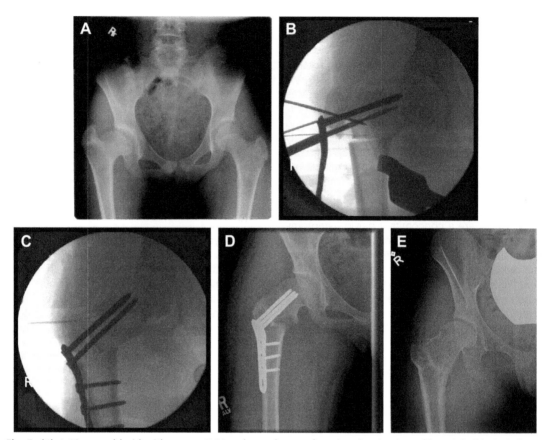

Fig. 5. (A) A 10-year-old girl with severe AVN and coxa breva after closed reduction of her right hip in infancy. She can walk only 100 m without severe pain, has 4 cm of shortening of her leg, and has a marked Trendelenburg gait. She has an excellent range of motion of her hip but signs of femoral-acetabular impingement. (B) An intra-operative image of a Wagner double osteotomy after lateral and distal transfer of the greater trochanter and fixation but before lateral and valgus displacement of the distal femur. (C) Intraoperative image of the completed osteotomy. Note the restoration of a normal neck-shaft angle and the tip of the greater trochanter at the level of the center of the femoral head. (D) The postoperative radiograph. (E) Note the remodeling of the proximal femur. She has no pain, can walk unlimited distances, and has a normal gait, excellent range of motion, a negative Trendelenburg test, and only 1.5 cm of shortening of the leg. A Ganz periacetabular osteotomy is planned to complete the reconstruction of her hip.

as combined or staged procedures, may be required to relieve pain, improve function, and delay the inevitable onset of degenerative arthritis. The choice of osteotomy must be made after careful clinical and radiographic evaluation of a patient, with the aim of providing an optimal biomechanical environment for the fragile hip. After the acetabular triradiate cartilage has closed, the pelvic osteotomy of choice is usually a Bernese periacetabular osteotomy, providing the hip is reasonably congruent and osteoarthritis has not advanced to the stage of marked loss of the joint cartilage space seen on plain radiographs. CT scanning is valuable in assessing the configuration of the acetabulum and femoral head. MRI is helpful in assessing the integrity of the articular cartilage of the hip joint.

Fig. 5 demonstrates the Wagner double osteotomy or femoral neck-lengthening osteotomy.[9] This is a useful technique for reconstructing the proximal femur in cases of severe late AVN, which aims to restore a normal biomechanical profile to the proximal femur in terms of femoral neck length, neck-shaft angle, and articulotrochanteric distance. The first osteotomy cut is at the base of the greater trochanter in line with the superior aspect of the neck of the femur and the second is perpendicular to the shaft of the femur at the level if the lesser trochanter. The greater trochanter is mobilized and displaced distally and laterally such that the tip of the trochanter is at the level of the center of the femoral head. The neck-shaft angle is corrected to 130° where necessary and the distal femoral shaft is displaced laterally. The osteotomies are fixed with a blade plate or a pediatric hip locking plate (see **Fig. 5**). The Morscher variant of this osteotomy[10] aims to achieve exactly the same goals as the Wagner osteotomy; however, it differs in that the distal osteotomy is oriented in line with the femoral neck at the desired neck-shaft angle, achieving a more direct neck and limb lengthening effect. The proximal osteotomy for greater trochanteric advancement also differs in that a cylinder of bone is removed at its base, again at the angle of the desired neck-shaft angle. A Morscher osteotomy, therefore, does not alter the orientation of the femoral head in the acetabulum, in contrast to the Wagner osteotomy. The benefits of the double osteotomy are partial restoration of leg length, improved abductor function, markedly improved gait, and correction of varus deformity, if present, all within one procedure.

More often than not a Bernese periacetabular osteotomy is also required to correct residual acetabular dysplasia, as seen in the patient illustrated in **Fig. 5**. This can be done simultaneously with the femoral double osteotomy but disturbs the abductor musculature at both the proximal and distal attachments, potentially compromising blood and nerve supply, and could place excessive tension on the abductor muscles and jeopardize the fixation of the greater trochanter. For these reasons, the authors prefer the pelvic osteotomy, if required, after union of the femoral osteotomy and recovery of the abductor muscle strength.

SUMMARY

The operative management of DDH is technically challenging. To achieve excellent results, surgeons need to select the most appropriate operative treatment, minimize the risk of complications, and be aggressive in the management of serious complications, such as redislocation and AVN, when they occur. We have described specific steps and strategies to assist in each of these key steps.

REFERENCES

1. Zionts LE, MacEwen GD. Treatment of congenital dislocation of the hip between the ages of one and three years. J Bone Joint Surg Am 1986;68: 829–46.
2. Agus A, Omeroglu H, Bicimoglu A, et al. Is Kalamchi and MacEwen group I avascular necrosis of the femoral head harmless in developmental dislocation of the hip? Hip Int 2010;20:156–62.
3. Morcuende JA, Meyer MD, Dolan LA, et al. Long-term outcome after open reduction through an anteromedial approach for congenital dislocation of the hip. J Bone Joint Surg Am 1997;79:810–7.
4. Roposch A, Liu LQ, Offiah AC, et al. Functional outcomes in children with osteonecrosis secondary to treatment of developmental dislocation of the hip. J Bone Joint Surg Am 2011;93:2263.
5. Thomas SR, Wedge JH, Salter RB. Outcome at forty-five years after open reduction and innominate osteotomy for late-presenting developmental dislocation of the hip. J Bone Joint Surg Am 2007;89: 2341–50.
6. Brougham DI, Broughton NS, Cole WG, et al. Avascular necrosis following closed reduction of congenital dislocation of the hip. Review of influencing factors and long-term follow-up. J Bone Joint Surg Br 1990;70:733–6.
7. Kalamchi A, MacEwen GD. Avascular necrosis following treatment of congenital dislocation of the hip. J Bone Joint Surg Am 1980;62:876–88.
8. Bucholz RW, Ogden JA. Patterns of ischemic necrosis of the proximal femur in nonoperatively treated congenital hip disease. St Louis (MO): CV Mosby Co; 1978. p. 43–63.
9. Wagner H. Femoral osteotomies for congenital hip dislocation. In: Weil UH, editor. Progress in orthopaedic surgery, vol. 2. Berlin: Springer-Verlag; 1978. p. 103–5.
10. Hasler CC, Morscher EW. Femoral neck lengthening osteotomy after growth disturbance of the proximal femur. J Paediatr Orthop B 1999;8: 271–5.

Surgical Treatment of Hip Dysplasia in Children and Adolescents

Bernd Bittersohl, MD[a], Harish S. Hosalkar, MD[a],
Dennis R. Wenger, MD[a,b,*]

KEYWORDS

- Hip dysplasia • Children • Surgical treatment • Acetabuloplasty

KEY POINTS

- Residual hip dysplasia, a well-known cause for early osteoarthritis (OA), is a relatively common disorder in children and adolescents.
- Three-dimensional imaging, including CT and MRI assessment has enhanced the diagnosis and treatment of patients with dysplasia by allowing clear identification of important pathomorphologic anatomy and cartilage degeneration.
- Treatment of residual hip dysplasia requires surgery with a goal of normalizing joint loading by increasing the contact area and improving the level arm of the hip to forestall the development of OA.
- Proper selection and performance of a corrective acetabular osteotomy and adjunctive procedures to provide a well-covered femoral head are prerequisites for a good clinical outcome and high survivorship of the hip.

INTRODUCTION

The human hip develops in utero and evolves to a large polyaxial stable joint that under ideal circumstances can last a lifetime. Unfortunately, both genetic and acquired factors can prevent this ideal circumstance, leading to hip dysplasia and early secondary degenerative arthritis.

Modern neonatal diagnostic methods have minimized the late diagnosis of hip dysplasia, with ultrasound, allowing treatment in the first months of life. Despite this progress, however, some patients end up with residual hip dysplasia, which requires surgical treatment in childhood or adolescence. The goal of surgery is to convert shear forces to compression forces (for which the articular cartilage is well-designed to withstand) (**Figs. 1** and **2**). Obviously, the earlier correction is provided, the greater the chance for normal development of the acetabulum and hip joint.

The goal of this article is to briefly describe the nature of residual hip dysplasia in childhood and adolescence and to present indications and methods for performing commonly used surgical procedures to correct hip dysplasia.

HISTORY AND PHYSICAL EXAMINATION

Initial assessment should focus on the patient history, symptomatology, activity level, and functional limitations, if any.

[a] Department of Orthopedic Surgery, Rady Children's Hospital San Diego, 3030 Children's Way, Suite 410, San Diego, CA 92123, USA; [b] Department of Orthopedic Surgery, Rady Children's Hospital San Diego/UCSD, 3030 Children's Way, Suite 410, San Diego, CA 92123, USA
* Corresponding author. Department of Orthopedic Surgery, Rady Children's Hospital San Diego/UCSD, 3030 Children's Way, Suite 410, San Diego, CA 92123.
E-mail address: dwenger@rchsd.org

Orthop Clin N Am 43 (2012) 301–315
doi:10.1016/j.ocl.2012.05.004

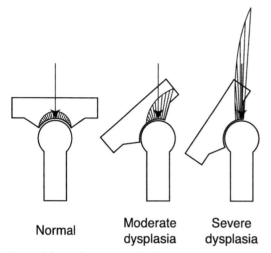

Normal   Moderate   Severe
dysplasia   dysplasia

Fig. 1. Schematic drawing clarifying how compression forces become shear forces in a patient with hip dysplasia. Concentration of forces on the acetabular rim leads to cartilage degeneration.

The history should include any pertinent risk factors, such as breech-presentation, high birth weight for gestational age, or oligohydraminios.[1] A family history of hip pathology should identify

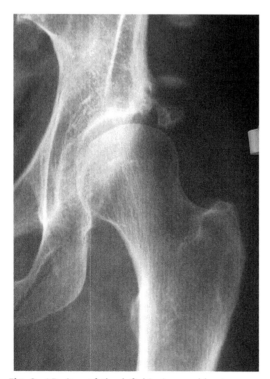

Fig. 2. AP view of the left hip in an older teenager with left hip dysplasia who now has severe pain. Concentration of forces on the anterolateral acetabular rim has led to a rim fracture, documenting the theory of Pauwels.

heredity factors, including a history of acetabular dysplasia and joint laxity in the family.[2] Parents of children with hip dysplasia/hip dislocation may have observed a variety of features in their child, such as limping, walking on tiptoe, difficulty in crawling, and asymmetry of thigh creases, hip abduction, or leg length.[3] Many children and adolescents are incidentally diagnosed following radiographs for other reasons and are asymptomatic.

Patients with residual dysplasia may be asymptomatic or experience slight discomfort with weight-bearing activities. Adolescents who additionally have a labral tear may experience catching or locking symptoms with occasional popping sensations in their hip joint. In older teenager and young adults, symptoms of continued pain should make the clinician suspect and evaluate for osteoarthritic (OA) changes. Finally, because dysplasia is often asymptomatic in the child and adolescent, many of the patients were treated or evaluated for hip dysplasia as infants and toddlers. Therefore, a detailed surgical history is often required.

EXAMINATION

Physical examination should include inspection of the extremities for limb-length discrepancy, angular or torsional malalignment of the limb, provocative testing for hip instability, and evaluation of hip motion, including assessment of difference in abduction. Gait analysis may reveal a very subtle limp in early childhood or Trendelenburg gait in an older child. Timed Trendelenburg test (10–20 seconds) allows for the assessment of relative abductor muscle weakness. Pelvic obliquity and spinal alignment for scoliosis should be tested. Pain elicited by hip flexion, adduction, and internal rotation (positive impingement test) can be potentially caused by a torn labrum or an acetabular rim syndrome, which is associated with a limbus or bone fragment that has detached from the rim of the acetabulum.[4] Of note, children with untreated hip dysplasia often have normal hip motion and no pain.[5]

IMAGING
Standard Radiography

Plain radiographic evaluation of hips aids in the comprehensive assessment of hip dysplasia, helps monitor hip development, may guide treatment, and also assists in assessment of treatment outcomes. This includes an anteroposterior (AP) pelvis and a lateral radiograph at a minimum.[5] A false- (faux-) profile image may be helpful in certain patients depending on their age and severity of dysplasia. Pelvic rotation and pelvic tilt should be considered for appropriate assessment of morphology.[6]

Several radiographic parametric indices are helpful in evaluating the skeletally immature hip,[7] including the Hilgenreiner line, the Perkins-Ombrédanne line (drawn at the lateral margin of the acetabulum perpendicular to the Hilgenreiner line), and the Shenton arc (line).

Further measurements can be performed to stratify or grade the severity of hip dysplasia, including the acetabular index,[8] Tonnis angle,[8] lateral center-edge angle (LCA) of Wiberg,[9] and, after fusion of the triradiate cartilage (in adults) the acetabular angle of Sharp.[10] The presence of a crossover sign[11] and a prominent ischial spine[12] are indicators for acetabular retroversion, which although rare, may be associated with hip dysplasia.

The false-(faux-) profile view as described by Lequesne and de Sèze[13] in 1961 allows for the assessment of the ventral center-edge angle (angle formed between a vertical line through the center of the femoral head and a line extending through the center of the femoral head to the anterior sourcil) as a potential determinant of the anterior acetabular coverage.

The appearance of the acetabular sourcil is a sensitive radiographic feature of symmetric or asymmetric loading of the hip joint.[14] This dense subchondral bone normally appears as a smooth curve with uniform thickness, forming the base of the so-called "Gothic Arch" with craniomedially and craniolaterally extending groups of trabeculae that meet above the sourcil to complete the arch. In the dysplastic hip, the sourcil appears tilted rather than level, and lateral sourcil thickening occurs, which represents increased focal loading related to the underlying malalignment of the joint.

Femoral torsion may be evaluated using a Dunn-Rippstein radiograph[15,16]; however, precise torsion profile assessment is feasible only by means of computed tomography (CT) or magnetic resonance (MR) imaging.

In older patients, radiographic examination of the hip joint in various positions can be valuable to evaluate the effect of a proposed osteotomy. For example, an abduction internal rotation radiograph reveals whether the femoral head can be concentrically reduced into the acetabulum. This view neutralizes femoral anteversion and allows accurate calculation of the femoral neck-shaft angle.

Acetabular dysplasia can be either associated with stable articulation or with articular instability including hip subluxation and hip dislocation. A patient with hip dysplasia has morphologic abnormalities of the acetabulum and/or femoral head with an intact Shenton line, whereas a patient with subluxation has anatomic abnormalities of the femoral head and/or acetabulum and a disruption of the Shenton line.

The long-term outcome after corrective hip osteotomy correlates with preexisting joint degeneration with less predictable findings in patients with preexisting OA changes. The degree of OA of the hip can be graded according to the Tönnis criteria[17]; however, detection of early cartilage changes, which is important for treatment and prognostication, remains a challenge and, as such, hip joint degeneration may be advanced by the time the diagnosis of OA is made based on plain radiography.

Advanced Imaging

Advanced imaging studies, such as MRI, MR arthrography, or CT examination with 3-dimensional (3D) reconstruction may be indicated in patients with severe hip dysplasia and/or patients who present late to (1) determine the exact location and character of the deformity, and (2) to reliably assess the status of hip joint structures (ie, cartilage and labrum), which is essential for surgical decision making, treatment planning, and prognostication.[18,19] The 3D evaluation provides superior information about the fit of the femoral head inside the acetabulum, as well as the size, shape, and orientation of both the acetabulum and femur (**Fig. 3**). Furthermore, CT or MRI examination, including torsional profile assessment may be indicated to define the exact degree of femoral and acetabular anteversion.[20,21]

With advances in hip preservation surgery, accurate assessment of joint cartilage status that includes detection of biochemical changes is becoming increasingly important (discussed in the article by Y.J. Kim, elsewhere in this issue).

SURGICAL TREATMENT—BASIC PRINCIPLES

In hip dysplasia, joint overloading occurs at the rim of a short and shallow acetabulum.[4] Two main components account for joint overloading: (1) increased muscle forces about the hip, and (2) decreased load-transferring weight-bearing surface area related to the shortness and obliquity of the dysplastic hip. Shear forces originating from the oblique acetabulum further contribute to lateralization of the hip joint center. Eventually, progressive cartilage degeneration associated with soft-tissue impairment, such as labral damage and degeneration, may develop.[4,22]

The goal of surgical treatment is to reduce the joint loading by increasing the contact area, relaxing the capsule and muscles about the hip, and improving the lever arm of the hip to restore hip

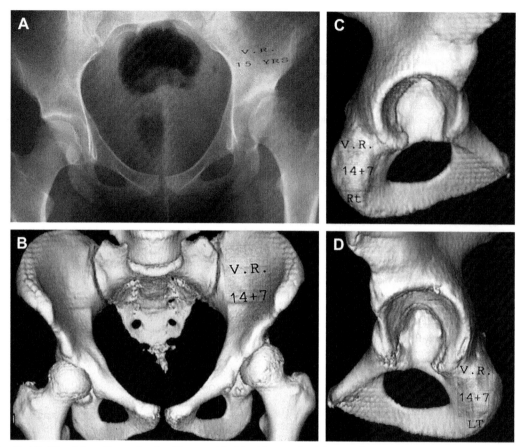

Fig. 3. (A) AP pelvis radiograph of a 15-year-old girl with no prior history who now has left hip pain. The films show acetabular dysplasia (*left*) with hip subluxation. (B) Anteroposterior 3D CT study of same patient. (C) Lateral 3D CT view of the more normal right hip acetabulum. (D) Lateral view of the dysplastic left acetabulum. Note the change in acetabular shape, demonstrating dysplasia.

biomechanics, provide joint stability, and potentially forestall the development of OA.[23,24] In infants and younger children, the restoration of hip-joint concentricity may set the stage for subsequent remodeling,[25] whereas relieving symptoms, maintaining or improving activity and quality of life, and delaying the total hip arthroplasty may be the more limited goal in patients with more severe hip dysplasia.

Many hip osteotomies and soft tissue procedures to accomplish these goals have been reported that vary depending on the patient's age, severity of dysplasia, morphology of the hip joint, coexisting soft tissue pathology, preexisting OA, and surgeon comfort. These procedures include femoral procedures, such as derotation, varization, and shortening femoral osteotomies, and pelvic osteotomies, such as Salter innominate osteotomy,[25] juxta-articular double osteotomy,[26] triple pelvis osteotomies,[27–29] periacetabular osteotomies (PAOs),[30] Pemberton pericapsular osteotomy,[31] and Dega transiliac osteotomy.[32]

Spherical osteotomies described by Wagner, Eppright, and others[33–35] may be used to cover severely dysplastic hips; however, these procedures are technically difficult and are prone to complications, such as inadvertent penetration of the acetabulum and/or avascular necrosis.

Age-Related Indications

Residual hip dysplasia can be a major cause of disability and is best corrected at an early age. Previous studies have demonstrated that early surgical correction of residual dysplasia will delay or prevent the onset of premature arthritis.[36,37] Furthermore, in younger children, residual hip dysplasia or subluxation may be more predictably corrected, with better clinical and radiographic results, less morbidity, and fewer complications.[38,39] However, the debate about the minimum age, at which a hip osteotomy should be performed remains controversial. On the assumption that the potential for acetabular remodeling is significantly reduced after the age of 18 months, Salter and coworkers proposed his procedure to be done after that age,[25,39] whereas others believe that pelvic osteotomy has limited indications in children younger than 5 years.[40]

Acetabular osteotomies are characterized as redirectional or reshaping procedures that are performed either as a reconstructive or a salvage procedure. Complete acetabular procedures, such as the Salter, triple pelvic (TPO), or Bernese PAO, improve the coverage of the femoral head by redirecting the acetabulum. The shape of the acetabulum itself remains unchanged. Reshaping osteotomies, such as the Pemberton or Dega osteotomy, change the shape of the acetabulum. Because redirectional procedures involve complete cuts through the innominate bone, fixation is required to maintain the new alignment until the osteotomy heals, whereas reshaping osteotomies in general do not require additional fixation.

The Salter single innominate osteotomy or reshaping procedures (ie, Pemberton or Dega osteotomy) may be used for dysplastic hips in younger children (younger than 8 or 9 years). In older children and adolescents, where the acetabulum may have to be displaced to a greater degree to provide sufficient coverage of the hip, procedures including the TPO and PAO are used. This article focuses on osteotomies (ie, Salter osteotomy, TPO) that do not cross the triradiate acetabular growth cartilage and can be used in the growing child. In contrast, the PAO (described in a later article in this issue) is performed in mature adolescents and young adults in whom the triradiate growth cartilage is closed.

Finally, the ability to concentrically reduce and maintain the femoral head within the acetabulum must be analyzed when surgical treatment is considered. In severe cases, a simultaneous femoral osteotomy may be needed.

Incongruent Hip Joint

Joints that are relatively incongruent and cannot be concentrically reduced, or those that reveal notable changes of degeneration, may benefit from "salvage" procedures, such as the Chiari osteotomy[41] or Staheli shelf procedure.[42] However, whereas reconstructive procedures have a relatively predictable outcome, the main expectation from any kind of salvage procedure is to help relieve pain, delay the inevitable hip arthroplasty, and possibly improve function in the meantime.

PROXIMAL FEMORAL OSTEOTOMY

A proximal femoral shortening osteotomy is commonly performed with primary hip dislocation to decrease the compressive forces on the femoral head after the reduction to potentially decrease the risk of avascular necrosis. When a child with hip dislocation is older than 2 years, a combined open reduction and acetabular procedure with a proximal femur osteotomy (varus derotation with/without shortening) may be performed.[43] In the past, proximal varus derotation osteotomy (which was acclaimed as a technically easier procedure as compared with pelvic osteotomy) was used in younger children with hip dysplasia with the consideration that concentric reduction served as the primary stimulus for acetabular remodeling.[44] Lalonde and colleagues[38] noted that isolated varus osteotomy was unpredictable for correcting hip dysplasia, even in children as young as 4 years.

Spence and colleagues[45] compared acetabular development in children of walking age managed for dislocation of the hip with open reduction combined with either a femoral varus derotation osteotomy or an innominate osteotomy, noting that acetabular remodeling after open hip reduction and innominate osteotomy was more effective for reversing acetabular dysplasia and maintaining hip stability than open reduction combined with a femoral varus derotation osteotomy.

In our current practice, we do not perform an isolated varus osteotomy to correct residual hip dysplasia in childhood. Femoral osteotomy is sometimes performed in combination with an acetabular procedure in cases of severe dysplasia with high subluxation.

REDIRECTIONAL ACETABULAR OSTEOTOMIES
Salter Innominate Osteotomy

Described by Salter in 1961,[25] the single innominate osteotomy was reported as a method to add immediate stability when reducing a completely dislocated hip in children older than 18 months (described in an earlier article in this issue). The Salter innominate osteotomy has also been commonly used to correct residual dysplasia in childhood up to about age 10 years. The procedure is widely used owing to its long track record and relative ease of performance (if the surgeon is properly trained).

The Salter procedure provides improved anterolateral coverage by redirecting the acetabulum without changing acetabular shape or volume (**Fig. 4**A). The primary indication for the Salter procedure is, therefore, deficiency in anterolateral coverage in an otherwise concentrically reduced hip in children between 2 and 10 years of age. The undersized acetabulum is redirected, avoiding

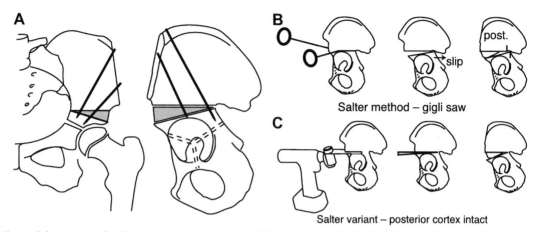

Fig. 4. (A) Conceptual Salter innominate osteotomy. (B) Standard method of making cut for the Salter innominate osteotomy using a Gigli saw. The complete cut may allow posterior displacement of the acetabular segments. This can occur even after pin fixation if the pins are not well placed. (C) Modified method for Salter osteotomy carefully using a saw and osteotome, with the cortex left intact in the sciatic notch. This prevents posterior displacement of the distal fragment and provides a more stable variant of the Salter procedure.

the risk of an acetabular bending procedure that might decrease the size or volume of the acetabulum. Depending on age and acetabular fragment mobility through the pliable fulcrum of the pubic symphysis, adequate improvement in the LCA as well the acetabular index may be expected.[46]

Children younger than 2 years may have inadequate iliac bone to support pin fixation, whereas in children older than 10 years, the decreased flexibility of the pubic symphysis prevents sufficient movement of the acetabular fragment. A steep, shallow elongated acetabulum is a relative contraindication and may be better treated with a reshaping procedure.

Procedure

The hip is approached through the anterolateral Smith-Peterson interval, which is, in the children's orthopedic world, usually referred to as the Salter approach. The inner and outer tables of the iliac wing are exposed subperiosteally and a straight osteotomy is made with a Gigli saw from the sciatic notch to the anterior-inferior iliac spine. Adequate exposure and proper subperiosteal clearing of the sciatic notch is required to prevent injuries of neurovascular structures.

The Salter procedure mildly increases limb length and also increases tension on the muscles that cross the hip anteriorly. Therefore, an iliopsoas intramuscular lengthening at the pelvic brim is performed to decrease compression on the femoral head and enhance distal fragment mobility.

The acetabular portion is pulled forward and rotated slightly anterolateral by rotating through the flexible fulcrum of the pubic symphysis with the proximal fragment held in place, leaving the

posterior site of the osteotomy closed. Inadvertent opening of the osteotomy posteriorly displaces the hip joint distally, resulting in leg lengthening and less acetabular coverage. A towel clamp placed in the iliac bone just above the acetabulum can be used as a handle to guide the displacement and rotation of the acetabulum.

If the capsule is intact, the displacement of the acetabular fragment may be further facilitated by placing the patient's leg into a figure-of-4 position (hip flexion, abduction, and external rotation) while being careful to prevent retroversion. In his description of the procedure, Salter emphasized that when the acetabular fragment is rotated forward, the anterior superior and inferior iliac spines should be kept aligned. Although the concept was not described as such, he meant "avoid creating acetabular retroversion"—a concept now well appreciated, as excessive acetabular retroversion can be a risk factor for early hip arthritis.

A triangular bone graft, taken from the anterior-superior iliac spine area, is placed into the osteotomy and the osteotomy is fixed with threaded K-wires. One pin directed behind the acetabulum and one superior and medial to the acetabulum transfix the bone graft. Image intensifier views ensure proper correction and fixation.

Postoperative treatment includes 6 weeks in a single hip spica cast followed by 3 additional weeks of partial weight-bearing.

Salter variant

Salter emphasized that the iliac osteotomy should be complete to allow sufficient anterior and lateral movement of the acetabulum; however, this mobility increases the risks associated with the procedure (ie, posterior slippage and loss of fixation) (see **Fig. 4**B).

Accordingly, when treating hip dysplasia alone (not in association with open reduction), we often use a power saw for the anterior two-thirds of the osteotomy cut and then an osteotome, cutting the bone to a point just anterior to the sciatic notch. The osteotomy is then hinged opened, leaving the posterior cortex intact. The bone graft and K-wire fixation are the same as in the traditional Salter procedure (see **Fig. 4**C). The result is a safe, stable Salter procedure with little risk for inadvertent displacement and/or loss of fixation.

Triple Pelvic Osteotomy

In older children (>8 years), hinging and rotation on the triradiate cartilage or pubic symphysis becomes more difficult because of skeletal maturity and decreased ligamentous laxity. One can still perform a Salter innominate osteotomy in this age group but dysplasia correction may be insufficient, especially in severe grades of dysplasia. Furthermore, potential upward migration and/or rotation of the proximal segment through the sacroiliac joint can lead to a loss of correction over time. Therefore, residual hip dysplasia in older children is managed better with a TPO. After closure of the triradiate cartilage, the Bernese PAO can be considered an alternative to the triple innominate osteotomy.

The TPO was first described by Steel,[28] but due to editorial dating errors by a journal, was attributed to Le Coeur.[47] Briefly summarized, the approach includes a transverse osteotomy of the ilium through a Smith-Peterson approach just above the acetabular roof and cutting of the superior and inferior pubic rami. The acetabulum was then rotated laterally and anteriorly to improve coverage of the femoral head.

Since then, several modifications of the original TPO, including the Tönnis[29] and the Carlioz[27] procedures, have been described; however, the principle of the triple innominate osteotomy remains the same: it involves osteotomies of the ischium and pubis in addition to the iliac osteotomy to allow free mobility and rotation of the acetabular fragment (**Fig. 5**).

Steel method
Steel's osteotomies through the ischial and pubis rami include a horizontal incision made over the ischial tuberosity for the ischial osteotomy (directed approximately 45° posterolaterally) with the patient in the supine position and the hip and knee joint flexed at 90°, and an anterior iliofemoral incision for the pubic osteotomy (directed

posteriorly and medially).[28] The iliac osteotomy is performed as in the Salter procedure.

The potential disadvantage of the Steel procedure includes that the ischial osteotomy is below the sacrotuberous and sacrospinous ligaments, potentially decreasing the ability to reorient the acetabulum, and a tendency for lateralization and retroversion, owing to the restraints imposed by the remaining intact sacrospinous and sacrotuberous ligaments. Also, the ischial cut is far from the acetabulum, leaving a lengthy segment of ischial bone attached to the acetabulum, making rotation more difficult. Furthermore, with marked rotation, muscle may enter the ischial osteotomy site, making pseudarthrosis more likely. Therefore, the Steel triple osteotomy may have some limitation in severe acetabular dysplasia that requires extensive acetabular reorientation.

Tönnis method
The unique feature of the Tönnis procedure is the location of the ischial osteotomy, which is performed directly from a posterior approach with the patient in the prone position.[29] The cut is located immediately behind and below the acetabulum and connects the sciatic notch with the obturator foramen closely proximal to the ischial spine. The acetabular cut can then be made proximal to both the sacrotuberous ligament and the sacrospinous ligament, allowing free acetabular rotation.

The pubic and iliac cuts (performed from anterior with the patient in supine position) are circular and parallel to the hip joint (perpendicular pubic cut and slightly curved orientated iliac cut, respectively). The advantages of the Tönnis procedure are that the length of the ischial cut allows continued bony contact even after excessive ventral rotation of the acetabulum, and, because the osteotomies are performed close to the acetabulum, greater freedom for lateral rotation and medial displacement of the acetabular fragment is allowed because of bypassing the restraining ligaments. Disadvantages include the complexity of the procedure and the proximity of the posterior ischial cut to the sciatic nerve, which is, therefore, at relatively high risk for inadvertent damage. Also, the separate posterior approach mandates repositioning of the patient during surgery.

Carlioz–San Diego method
The San Diego approach represents a modification of the Carlioz procedure[27] in which the ischial cut is made just below the acetabulum and, then, directed horizontally between the sacrospinous and sacrotuberous ligaments (**Fig. 6**).[48] As in the Tönnis procedure, all cuts are made near the acetabulum, facilitating acetabular rotation;

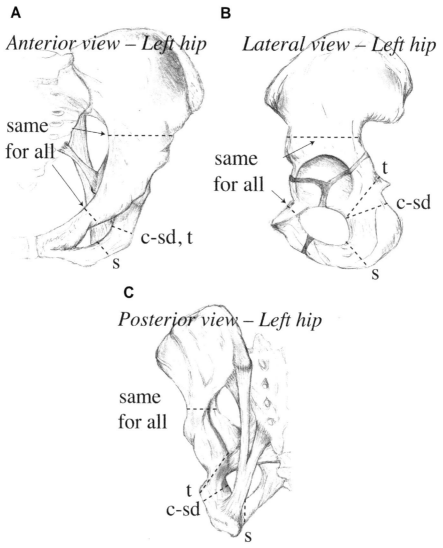

A

Anterior view – Left hip

same for all

c-sd, t

s

B

Lateral view – Left hip

same for all

t

c-sd

s

C

Posterior view – Left hip

same for all

t

c-sd

s

Fig. 5. Conceptual different types of triple pelvic osteotomy. The anterior (*A*), lateral (*B*), and posterior (*C*) views demonstrate the location of 3 osteotomy cuts for the Steel (s), Carlioz-San Diego (c-sd), and Tonnis (t) methods.

however, with our approach a separate posterolateral incision (required with the Tönnis technique) is avoided.

We perform the TPO in the following sequence: (1) iliac osteotomy, (2) pubic osteotomy, and (3) ischial osteotomy.[49] Therefore, a standard anterolateral incision for the iliac cut (identical to the Salter procedure) is made for the iliac osteotomy.

A small transverse incision in the medial groin (just below the pubis) is made for the pubic cut (superior pubic ramus). The pectineus muscle is identified and retracted inferiorly with subperiosteal dissection performed to expose the superior pubic ramus. An osteotome or rongeur is used to make the pubic cut.

With the hip flexed above 90°, the ischium can be approached either by extending the same

medial incision posterolaterally or by making a third separate longitudinal incision over the tip of the ischium. Soft tissue dissection includes detaching the adductor magnus origin to expose the ischium just below the acetabulum. The ischial cut is made 1 to 2 cm below the acetabulum, using a long osteotome.

Once the acetabulum is mobilized, the acetabular fragment is rotated anteriorly (sagittal plane) and laterally (coronal plane) to provide anterolateral coverage of the femoral head. This allows free rotation in which the Kohler tear drop is elevated rather than a pure hinging/rotation procedure, which occurs during the Salter procedure. If the ischial osteotomy is performed obliquely from lateral to medial, the acetabular fragment can be displaced medially, centering the hip center in

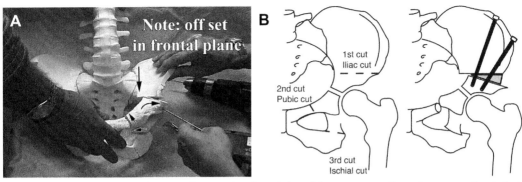

Fig. 6. (*A*) Schematic concept of acetabular rotation for triple pelvic osteotomy. The primary rotation is in the frontal plane. The 3 separate bone cuts adjacent to the acetabulum allow relatively free rotation of the acetabular fragment. (*B*) Preoperative and postoperative diagrams showing the sequence and level of cuts using the Carlioz-San Diego method of triple pelvic osteotomy.

the optimal physiologic position and improving gait mechanics.

A temporary large Schanz screw can be placed in the acetabular fragment and used as a handle to displace and guide the acetabulum. Care must be taken to bring the acetabulum forward and to rotate it in the frontal plane, avoiding external rotation at the same time . We do not recommend performing the "figure-of-4" procedure (as described by Salter to mobilize his osteotomy), because the greater instability produced by 3 cuts around the acetabulum may lead to undesirable external rotation and inadvertent retroversion of the acetabulum.

Care must also be undertaken to ensure that soft tissue (ie, muscle) does not intervene in the pubic and ischial cuts, which may lead to pseudarthrosis. Placement of bone graft and fixation of the pubic osteotomy is similar as for the Salter innominate procedure. Occasionally, screw fixation of the superior pubic ramus, as described by Tonnis and colleagues,[29] or plate fixation may be added to provide additional stability and minimize the risk for iatrogenic acetabular retroversion. Appropriate acetabular rotation, femoral head coverage, and osteotomy fixation are confirmed using the image intensifier. Postoperative care often includes a hip spica cast for 6 weeks followed by protected toe-touch weight-bearing for additional 6 weeks.

Periacetabular Osteotomy–Bernese PAO

The Bernese PAO originally described by Ganz and colleagues[30] in 1988 allows extensive acetabular reorientation including medial displacement to improve femoral head coverage and normalize loading of the anterolateral acetabular rim and is described in a later article in this issue. The procedure is sometimes used in adolescents older than 11 years when the triradiate cartilage is nearly

closed. One major benefit of the procedure is its innate stability, because no complete cut is made into the sciatic notch. Therefore, a postoperative cast is not required.

RESHAPING ACETABULAR PROCEDURES
Pemberton Acetabuloplasty

The pericapsular acetabuloplasty, as described by Pemberton in 1965,[31] hinges and rotates the acetabulum anteriorly and laterally through the posterior limb of the triradiate cartilage to improve coverage of the femoral head. An open triradiate cartilage is required for performing this procedure.

With angular hinging through the triradiate cartilage, acetabular shape can be changed, making this procedure especially suitable for cases in which the acetabulum is steep, capacious, and shallow (**Fig. 7**). On the other hand, the procedure is not recommended if the acetabulum is small relative to the size of the femoral head, as the reshaping decreases the size of the acetabular radius, which may prevent proper seating of the femoral head within the acetabulum.

The curvilinear cut begins anteriorly at the anterior-inferior iliac spine and proceeds posteriorly and inferiorly toward the posterior arm of the triradiate cartilage behind the acetabulum. The osteotomy includes both the outer and the inner wall of the ilium. By opening the osteotomy, the acetabular fragment is placed into an anterolateral position. A curvilinear triangular bone wedge taken from the iliac crest is firmly impacted into the osteotomy to hold the acetabulum in place. Internal fixation is normally not required, avoiding a potential operation for implant removal because the cut through the ilium is incomplete. On occasion, the osteotomy seems slightly unstable. In such cases, a single-threaded K-wire should be

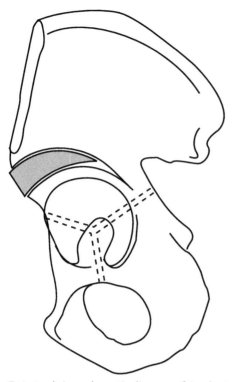

Fig. 7. Lateral view schematic diagram of Pemberton-type acetabuloplasty to correct hip dysplasia.

considered. Because the iliac cut is incomplete, bilateral Pemberton procedures can be performed on the same day.

Dega Acetabuloplasty

The transiliac osteotomy as described by Dega[32] starts anteriorly at the anterior-inferior iliac spine and extents posteriorly ending anterior to the sciatic notch (**Fig. 8**). The biomechanics and location of acetabular rotation appears to be almost identical to the Pemberton procedure.

Under image intensifier control, the osteotomy is directed toward the triradiate cartilage in a gently curved manner. The inner cortex of the ilium is preserved in this procedure. By opening the osteotomy with osteotomes, the acetabulum is pried inferiorly and laterally through the open triradiate cartilage. Triangular bone wedges either obtained from the femoral varization osteotomy (the Dega acetabuloplasty is often performed in combination with a proximal femoral varization osteotomy) or from the iliac crest are used to maintain the correction.

As in the Pemberton acetabuloplasty, the hinging forms a horizontal, arch-shaped acetabular surface, which makes this procedure suitable for cases in which the acetabulum is steep, capacious, and shallow.

San Diego Acetabuloplasty

The San Diego acetabuloplasty was originally described in 1992 as a modification of the Dega procedure, designed to provide improved coverage for patients with neuromuscular disease and hip dysplasia who have superoposterior acetabular deficiency.[50] Owing to objections from the "Dega community" and with further analysis, however, the San Diego acetabuloplasty has been more clearly defined. We refer to the procedure as a "spherical hinged acetabuloplasty" in which 3 triangular bone grafts are placed directly laterally with a primary goal of improving straight lateral and posterior-lateral acetabular deficiency (**Fig. 9**). We use the procedure almost exclusively for hip dysplasia in cerebral palsy and other neuromuscular conditions, where the acetabular deficiency has been documented to be superior and superior-posterior.[18]

The acetabular osteotomy begins anteriorly at the anterior-inferior iliac spine approximately 1 cm superior to the lateral margin of the acetabulum and proceeds in line to the sciatic notch, penetrating the outer wall of the ilium only, exact for the very anterior and posterior ends of the cut where a bicortical cut is made.

A straight or slightly curved osteotome is directed toward the medial aspect of the triradiate cartilage, preserving the joint and the inner wall of the pelvis. The osteotomy ends several millimeters above the triradiate cartilage to decrease the risk for potential damage to the triradiate cartilage and possible subsequent physeal closure.

Bicortical cuts are made both anteriorly over the anterior inferior iliac spine and posteriorly at the sciatic notch (in contrast to the Dega acetabuloplasty). This important step allows symmetric lateral and inferior hinging and lateral rotation of the acetabulum on or slightly above the triradiate cartilage to correct the dysplasia and produce a horizontal curve-shaped sourcil. Triangular bone wedges are harvested from the anterior crest of the ilium and placed into the osteotomy posteriorly, centrally, and anteriorly. The elasticity of the intact medial cortex predictably holds the bone grafts in place and internal fixation is not required. This procedure allows for sufficient posterior and superior coverage and can be used in any patient who has dysplasia and a true lateral acetabular deficiency (or the superior and posterior deficiency often seen in patients with cerebral palsy[18]).

SALVAGE PROCEDURES

Salvage procedures are designed to relieve pain, delay the inevitable hip arthroplasty, and improve function in the meantime. Hence, they remain

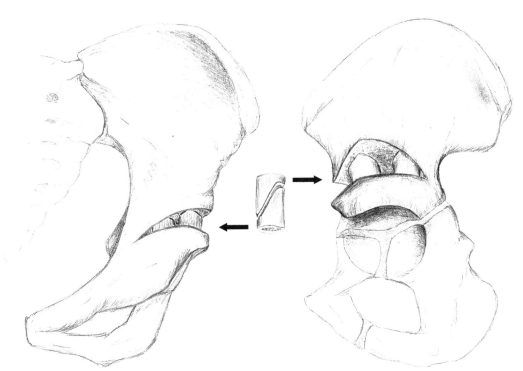

Fig. 8. Schematic diagram of AP and lateral pelvis demonstrating the original Dega-type corrective acetabulo-plasty. This method was designed to treat patients with a completely dislocated hip. A piece of the femur, which had been removed to shorten the femur to provide ease of reduction, is cut obliquely, providing 2 grafts to hold the osteotomy site open. The concept is similar to that of the Pemberton procedure.

potential treatment alternatives in residual hip dysplasia, in which a concentric reduction of the femoral head is technically not feasible and/or where advanced imaging assessment demonstrates severe, irreversible cartilage degeneration. Common examples of such procedures include

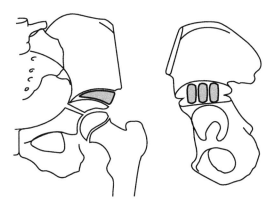

Fig. 9. Schematic San Diego acetabuloplasty designed to correct neuromuscular hip dysplasia. This spherical hinged acetabuloplasty cuts through both cortices (anteriorly at the level of the anterior inferior spine, posteriorly in the sciatic notch) but does not cross the medial cortex. Triangular grafts taken from the iliac crest are then inserted to hold the osteotomy open. This provides a very stable construct.

the Chiari osteotomy[41] and the Staheli slotted acetabular augmentation.[42]

The principle of these procedures is to gain coverage either by displacing (Chiari osteotomy) or by adding (slotted acetabular augmentation) bone of the ilium laterally over the femoral head. The hip capsule, which is buttressed by the displaced bone, is assumed to undergo gradual metaplasia to fibrocartilage that remodels with time to conform to the femoral head. With regard to the Chiari procedure, in addition to widening the contact area of the femoral head, the hip joint is displaced medially, further reducing the workload of the hip.

Chiari Osteotomy

The Chiari procedure is performed through an anterolateral approach, with the inner and outer tables of the ilium exposed to the sciatic notch.[41] The ilium cut begins anteriorly just above the acetabulum between the insertion of the capsule and the reflected tendon of the rectus and follows the capsular insertion in a slightly curved line to the sciatic notch posteriorly (**Fig. 10**).

The osteotomy is then completed by directing the cut medially and superiorly. Both starting point and slope of the osteotomy are critical and must

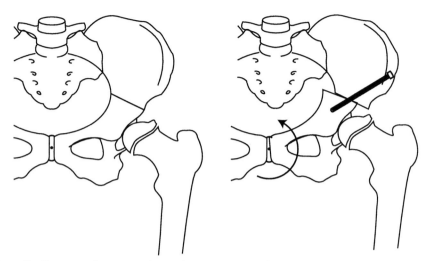

Fig. 10. Schematic diagrams of preoperative and postoperative Chiari osteotomy. Medial displacement of the acetabular segment allows the femoral head to be covered with hip capsule, which can develop into fibrocartilage. This is considered a salvage procedure for hip joints with significant incongruity.

be planned with caution to avoid impingement on the femoral head when it is displaced medially. For example, an osteotomy that starts too high, or where the angle of inclination is too horizontal, will not support the femoral head; whereas, if the slope of the osteotomy is too steep, the fragment will abut against the femoral head. In addition, an osteotomy, which enters the sacroiliac joint, cannot be displaced.

The amount of coverage that can maximally be obtained depends on the width of the ilium. The acetabular fragment must often be displaced medially almost the full width of the ilium to provide adequate lateral coverage. A bone graft taken from the iliac wing can be placed anteriorly over the femoral head if anterior coverage is inadequate after displacement of the osteotomy. The osteotomy is held in place with either pin or screw fixation once the translation of the iliac wing (lateral) and the acetabular fragment (medial) reveals sufficient coverage of the femoral head. A hip spica cast for 4 to 6 weeks may be applied to provide further stability until bone healing has occurred.

Slotted Acetabular Augmentation (Shelf Augmentation)

Numerous shelf procedures have been described[9,42,51–54]; however, the principle in these various forms remains the same: an extra-articular buttress (augmentation) is created, preventing further subluxation while potentially increasing the load-bearing area of the hip.[55] Shelf procedures are, like the Chiari osteotomy, salvage procedures, as they use bone over capsule to possibly stimulate fibrocartilage metaplasia rather than articular cartilage to increase the weight-bearing area. These procedures are indicated only when a congruent reduction is not feasible and/or when additional augmentation is required (ie, after other procedures, such as the Chiari osteotomy).

The slotted-shelf technique described by Staheli in 1981[56] (**Fig. 11**) is performed through an anterior iliofemoral approach exposing the outer wall of the ilium and the entire superior capsule of the hip joint. During this step, the reflected head of the rectus femoris is sectioned at its anterior part and dissected free from the capsule.

An approximately 1-cm-deep slot along the superior edge of the acetabulum is created and continued anteriorly and posteriorly as needed to provide the necessary coverage. The floor of the slot should exactly level with the insertion of the capsule. A series of drill holes and a narrow rongeur to connect these holes may be used to create the proper slot.

Several thin corticocancellous strips are then harvested from the outer table of the ilium and placed with the concave side facing downward radially into the slot. The strips are cut in proper length to add the desired amount of lateral coverage. Care must be taken to keep the lateral overhang of the bone grafts at an appropriate length, because this may lead to limited range of motion secondary to femoroacetabular impingement. A second layer of cancellous strips is placed lengthwise. Both layers are held in place by reattaching the tendon of the reflected head of the rectus femoris in its original position across the

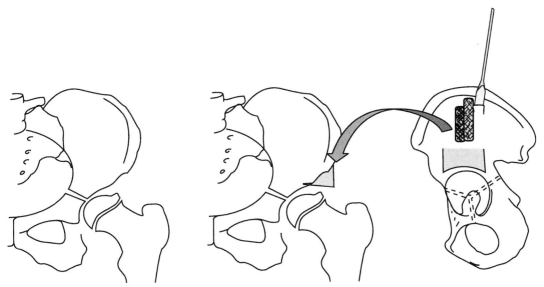

Fig. 11. Drawings demonstrating the principles of the Staheli shelf acetabuloplasty. The first figure shows a dysplastic hip with an incongruent femoral head. The second and third figures conceptually illustrate the procedure, and demonstrate how acetabular coverage can be improved. This procedure is used when there is an incongruous hip joint and is considered a salvage procedure.

graft. The remaining pieces of cancellous bone are packed over the reflected head of the rectus femoris, which are held in place by reattaching the hip abductor to the iliac crest, to further reinforce the shelf.

It is postulated that the shelf will gradually hypertrophy and remodel according to the pressure of the femoral head, whereas the capsule tissue will ideally transform into fibrocartilage tissue.

SUMMARY

Residual hip dysplasia (a relatively common condition in young children and adolescents) left undetected or partially treated, almost certainly leads to further progression of deformity, eventually ending in a nonfunctional, painful hip joint. Therefore, every effort should be made to identify and treat hip dysplasia early.

The use of 3D imaging, including CT and MRI assessment, has enhanced the diagnosis and treatment of patients with dysplasia because they facilitate proper identification of important pathomorphologic anatomy and cartilage degeneration. Future studies should take these novel imaging modalities into consideration with the attempt to (re-) evaluate optimal selection criteria for surgery, risk factors for clinical failure and optimal deformity correction.

Treatment of residual hip dysplasia requires corrective surgery. The goal of surgical treatment is to normalize joint loading by increasing the contact area and improving the level arm of the

hip to forestall the development of OA. Proper selection and performance of a correction osteotomy and adjunctive procedures are prerequisites for a good clinical outcome and high survivorship of the reconstructed hip.

Augmentation procedures, such as the Chiari osteotomy or the shelf procedure described by Staheli,[56] remain as a salvage option in cases when irreversible cartilage damage is present or when reorientation is not feasible.

REFERENCES

1. Chan A, McCaul KA, Cundy PJ, et al. Perinatal risk factors for developmental dysplasia of the hip. Arch Dis Child Fetal Neonatal Ed 1997;76(2):F94–100.
2. Wynne-Davies R. Acetabular dysplasia and familial joint laxity: two etiological factors in congenital dislocation of the hip. A review of 589 patients and their families. J Bone Joint Surg Br 1970;52(4):704–16.
3. David TJ, Parris MR, Poynor MU, et al. Reasons for late detection of hip dislocation in childhood. Lancet 1983;2(8342):147–9.
4. Klaue K, Durnin CW, Ganz R. The acetabular rim syndrome. A clinical presentation of dysplasia of the hip. J Bone Joint Surg Br 1991;73(3):423–9.
5. Weinstein SL, Mubarak SJ, Wenger DR. Developmental hip dysplasia and dislocation: Part I. Instr Course Lect 2004;53:523–30.
6. Tannast M, Zheng G, Anderegg C, et al. Tilt and rotation correction of acetabular version on pelvic radiographs. Clin Orthop Relat Res 2005;438: 182–90.

7. Hak DJ, Gautsch TL. A review of radiographic lines and angles used in orthopedics. Am J Orthop (Belle Mead NJ) 1995;24(8):590–601.

8. Tonnis D. Congenital dysplasia and dislocation of the hip in children and adults. Berlin: Springer; 1987.

9. Wiberg G. Shelf operation in congenital dysplasia of the acetabulum and in subluxation and dislocation of the hip. J Bone Joint Surg Am 1953;35(1):65–80.

10. Sharp IK. Acetabular dysplasia: the acetabular angle. J Bone Joint Surg Br 1961;43:268–72.

11. Jamali AA, Mladenov K, Meyer DC, et al. Antero-posterior pelvic radiographs to assess acetabular retroversion: high validity of the "cross-over-sign". J Orthop Res 2007;25(6):758–65.

12. Kalberer F, Sierra RJ, Madan SS, et al. Ischial spine projection into the pelvis: a new sign for acetabular retroversion. Clin Orthop Relat Res 2008;466(3): 677–83.

13. Lequesne M, de Sèze. False profile of the pelvis. A new radiographic incidence for the study of the hip. Its use in dysplasias and different coxopathies. Rev Rhum Mal Osteoartic 1961;28:643–52 [in French].

14. Pauwels F, Furlong RJ, Maquet P. Biomechanics of the normal and diseased hip: theoretical foundation, technique and results of treatment—an atlas. New York: Springer; 1976.

15. Dunn DM. Anteversion of the neck of the femur; a method of measurement. J Bone Joint Surg Br 1952;34(2):181–6.

16. Rippstein J. Determination of the antetorsion of the femur neck by means of two x-ray pictures. Z Orthop Ihre Grenzgeb 1955;86(3):345–60 [in German].

17. Tonnis D. Normal values of the hip joint for the evaluation of x-rays in children and adults. Clin Orthop Relat Res 1976;(119):39–47.

18. Kim HT, Wenger DR. Location of acetabular deficiency and associated hip dislocation in neuromuscular hip dysplasia: three-dimensional computed tomographic analysis. J Pediatr Orthop 1997;17(2): 143–51.

19. Kim YJ, Jaramillo D, Millis MB, et al. Assessment of early osteoarthritis in hip dysplasia with delayed gadolinium-enhanced magnetic resonance imaging of cartilage. J Bone Joint Surg Am 2003;85(10): 1987–92.

20. Hernandez RJ, Poznanski AK. CT evaluation of pediatric hip disorders. Orthop Clin North Am 1985; 16(3):513–41.

21. Koenig JK, Pring ME, Dwek JR. MR evaluation of femoral neck version and tibial torsion. Pediatr Radiol 2012;42(1):113–5.

22. Jessel RH, Zurakowski D, Zilkens C, et al. Radiographic and patient factors associated with pre-radiographic osteoarthritis in hip dysplasia. J Bone Joint Surg Am 2009;91(5):1120–9.

23. Albinana J, Dolan LA, Spratt KF, et al. Acetabular dysplasia after treatment for developmental dysplasia of the hip. Implications for secondary procedures. J Bone Joint Surg Br 2004;86(6):876–86.

24. Brand RA. Hip osteotomies: a biomechanical consideration. J Am Acad Orthop Surg 1997;5(5): 282–91.

25. Salter RB. Innominate osteotomy in the treatment of congenital hip dislocation and subluxation of the hip. J Bone Joint Surg Br 1961;43:518–39.

26. Sutherland DH, Moore M. Clinical and radiographic outcome of patients treated with double innominate osteotomy for congenital hip dysplasia. J Pediatr Orthop 1991;11(2):143–8.

27. Carlioz H, Khouri N, Hulin P. Triple juxtacotyloid osteotomy. Rev Chir Orthop Reparatrice Appar Mot 1982;68(7):497–501 [in French].

28. Steel HH. Triple osteotomy of the innominate bone. J Bone Joint Surg Am 1973;55(2):343–50.

29. Tonnis D, Behrens K, Tscharani F. A modified technique of the triple pelvic osteotomy: early results. J Pediatr Orthop 1981;1(3):241–9.

30. Ganz R, Klaue K, Vinh TS, et al. A new periacetabular osteotomy for the treatment of hip dysplasias. Technique and preliminary results. Clin Orthop Relat Res 1988;(232):26–36.

31. Pemberton PA. Pericapsular osteotomy of the ilium for treatment of congenital subluxation and dislocation of the hip. J Bone Joint Surg Am 1965;47: 65–86.

32. Dega W. Transiliac osteotomy in the treatment of congenital hip dysplasia. Chir Narzadow Ruchu Ortop Pol 1974;39(5):601–13 [in Polish].

33. Eppright RH. Dial osteotomy in the treatment of dysplasia of the hip. Paper presented at: Proceedings of the American Orthopaedic Association. 1975.

34. Ninomiya S, Tagawa H. Rotational acetabular osteotomy for the dysplastic hip. J Bone Joint Surg Am 1984;66(3):430–6.

35. Wagner H. Experiences with spherical acetabular osteotomy for the correction of the dysplastic acetabulum. Berlin: Springer; 1978.

36. Gillingham BL, Sanchez AA, Wenger DR. Pelvic osteotomies for the treatment of hip dysplasia in children and young adults. J Am Acad Orthop Surg 1999;7(5):325–37.

37. Harris NH. Acetabular growth potential in congenital dislocation of the hip and some factors upon which it may depend. Clin Orthop Relat Res 1976;(119): 99–106.

38. Lalonde FD, Frick SL, Wenger DR. Surgical correction of residual hip dysplasia in two pediatric age-groups. J Bone Joint Surg Am 2002; 84(7):1148–56.

39. Salter RB, Dubos JP. The first fifteen years' personal experience with innominate osteotomy in the

treatment of congenital dislocation and subluxation of the hip. Clin Orthop Relat Res 1974;(98):72–103.

40. Lindstrom JR, Ponseti IV, Wenger DR. Acetabular development after reduction in congenital dislocation of the hip. J Bone Joint Surg Am 1979;61(1):112–8.

41. Chiari K. Medial displacement osteotomy of the pelvis. Clin Orthop Relat Res 1974;(98):55–71.

42. Staheli LT, Chew DE. Slotted acetabular augmentation in childhood and adolescence. J Pediatr Orthop 1992;12(5):569–80.

43. Wenger DR. Congenital hip dislocation: techniques for primary open reduction including femoral shortening. Instr Course Lect 1989;38:343–54.

44. Schoenecker PL, Anderson DJ, Capelli AM. The acetabular response to proximal femoral varus rotational osteotomy. Results after failure of post-reduction abduction splinting in patients who had congenital dislocation of the hip. J Bone Joint Surg Am 1995;77(7):990–7.

45. Spence G, Hocking R, Wedge JH, et al. Effect of innominate and femoral varus derotation osteotomy on acetabular development in developmental dysplasia of the hip. J Bone Joint Surg Am 2009;91(11):2622–36.

46. Utterback JD, MacEwen GD. Comparison of pelvic osteotomies for the surgical correction of the congenital hip. Clin Orthop Relat Res 1974;(98):104–10.

47. Le Coeur P. Correction des défauts d'orientation de l'isthme iliaque. Rev Chir Orthop 1965;51:211–2.

48. Aminian A, Mahar A, Yassir W, et al. Freedom of acetabular fragment rotation following three surgical techniques for correction of congenital deformities of the hip. J Pediatr Orthop 2005;25(1):10–3.

49. Wenger DR, Pring ME. Triple innominate osteotomy. In: Wiesel S, editor. Operative techniques in orthopedic surgery, vol. 2. Philadelphia: Lippincott Williams & Wilkins; 2011. p. 1540–51.

50. Mubarak SJ, Valencia FG, Wenger DR. One-stage correction of the spastic dislocated hip. Use of pericapsular acetabuloplasty to improve coverage. J Bone Joint Surg Am 1992;74(9):1347–57.

51. Albee FH. Orthopedic and reconstruction surgery. Philadelphia: WB Saunders Co; 1919.

52. König F. Bildung einer knöchernen Hemmung für den Gelenkkopf bei der kongenitalen Luxation. Zentralbl Chir 1891;17:146–7.

53. Love BR, Stevens PM, Williams PF. A long-term review of shelf arthroplasty. J Bone Joint Surg Br 1980;62(3):321–5.

54. Nishimatsu H, Iida H, Kawanabe K, et al. The modified Spitzy shelf operation for patients with dysplasia of the hip. A 24-year follow-up study. J Bone Joint Surg Br 2002;84(5):647–52.

55. Bowen JR, Guille JT, Jeong C, et al. Labral support shelf arthroplasty for containment in early stages of Legg-Calve-Perthes disease. J Pediatr Orthop 2011;31(Suppl 2):S206–11.

56. Staheli LT. Slotted acetabular augmentation. J Pediatr Orthop 1981;1(3):321–7.

Surgery for Residual Femoral Deformity in Adolescents

Dror Paley, MD, FRCSC*

KEYWORDS

- Coxa valga • Coxa vara • Intertrochanteric osteotomy • Relative neck lengthening
- Trochanteric overgrowth

KEY POINTS

- Proximal femoral deformity and hip dysplasia are interrelated: proximal femoral deformity can affect the final shape of the acetabulum.
- Although there has been a recent emphasis on femoral head shape and head/neck offset abnormalities, the neck shaft angle, medial proximal femoral angle, femoral neck length, and greater and lesser trochanter position are important factors when addressing hip dysplasia.
- Anatomic abnormalities of the proximal femur have an effect on abductor and hip flexor muscle function and strength.
- There are many surgical options to normalize proximal femoral anatomy that should be considered when treating hip dysplasia. Proper analysis of the abnormal geometry of the bony femur, as well as the abnormal lever arms around the hip related to the lesser and greater trochanteric positions, is an essential part of a successful surgical plan.

INTRODUCTION

Femoral deformity and acetabular dysplasia are often associated with each other. Femoral deformity can be secondary to primary hip dysplasia and hip dysplasia can be secondary to primary femoral deformity,[1] because the forces of the femoral head on the acetabulum are integral to the development of acetabular depth and version and, conversely, the forces of the acetabulum on the femoral head are integral to the development of femoral neck inclination and version. The shape of the upper femur is also affected by any imbalance of muscle forces around it, such as from spasticity (cerebral palsy), paralysis (polio, Charcot Marie-Tooth) or even subtle neurologic disorders (eg, congenital pseudarthrosis with neurofibromatosis). This change in shape of the upper femur may lead to secondary dysplasia of the acetabulum (Fig. 1). Coxa valga produces lateral and superior forces on the acetabulum, eventually leading to

dysplasia.[1] Anteversion of the femur similarly leads to less medial force on the acetabulum and creates an apparent coxa valga. Furthermore, the posterior location of the greater trochanter in the anteverted femur decreases the abductor muscle lever arm, decreasing the medial force on the acetabulum and promoting hip dysplasia.[2] Acetabular dysplasia is often associated with femoral anteversion. Did the anteversion cause the dysplasia; did the dysplasia cause the anteversion; or are they both primary deformities associated with each other? The answer to this chicken-and-egg question remains unknown.

Coxa vara promotes increased medial forces on the hip and therefore better acetabular development. In soft bone diseases, coxa vara leads to coxa profunda and protrusio.[1] Therefore, when coxa vara is seen with hip dysplasia, it is not the cause of the dysplasia. The likelihood is that both deformities developed as part of the original disease process. Examples of coxa vara with

Paley Advanced Limb Lengthening Institute, Kimmel Building, St Mary's Hospital, 901 45th Street, West Palm Beach, FL 33407, USA
* Corresponding author.
E-mail address: dpaley@lengthening.us

Orthop Clin N Am 43 (2012) 317–328
doi:10.1016/j.ocl.2012.05.009
0030-5898/12/$ – see front matter © 2012 Elsevier Inc. All rights reserved.

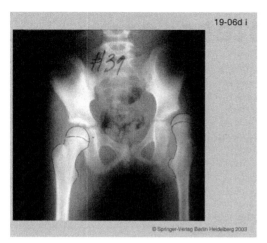

19-06d i

© Springer-Verlag Berlin Heidelberg 2003

Fig. 1. Severe valgus deformity of the femoral neck secondary to neurofibromatosis and congenital pseudarthrosis of the tibia. The acetabulum is becoming dysplastic and the femoral head is subluxating laterally. (*From* Paley D. Principles of deformity correction. 1st edition, 3rd printing. Berlin: Springer-Verlag; 2005; with permission.)

hip dysplasia are congenital coxa vara, congenital femoral deficiency, and Conradi-Hünermann syndrome.

Femoral deformities can also arise secondary to the treatment of hip dysplasia. For example, avascular necrosis of the proximal femur that occurs following nonoperative or operative treatment can produce a growth arrest of the upper femoral growth plate with either varus or valgus deformity of the femoral head on the femoral neck. Most of these cases do not manifest damage to the greater

trochanteric apophysis and therefore there is significant overgrowth of the greater trochanter. Growth arrest also leads to coxa breva, which alters the abductor and psoas tendon lever arms. Avascular necrosis can also lead to deformity of the femoral head, resulting in coxa magna or elliptical or saddle-shaped femoral head.

Evaluation of Femoral Deformities Associated with Hip Dysplasia

The history and physical examination are important in the evaluation of deformities around the hip. This evaluation should include the hip range of motion, presence or absence of impingement, rotation profile of the femur and tibia, and hip flexion and abduction strength and pain.

Plain radiographs still provide most of the information needed. Abduction and adduction views are also helpful. Computerized tomography is especially useful to evaluate the shape of the femoral head and acetabulum. Magnetic resonance arthrography is useful to evaluate for labral abnormality and impingement.

The joint orientation angles of the hip and knee in the frontal plane should be evaluated (medial proximal femoral angle [MPFA] and neck shaft angle [NSA] for both hips, and lateral distal femoral angle [LDFA] and medial proximal tibial angle [MPTA] for the knee). The difference between the MPFA of both hips should be compared with the difference between the NSA for both hips. If the differences are the same, then there is no trochanteric overgrowth. If the differences are different, then there is trochanteric overgrowth (**Figs. 2–4**).[2]

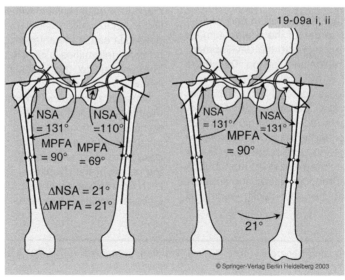

19-09a i, ii

NSA = 131°   NSA =110°
MPFA = 90°   MPFA = 69°
ΔNSA = 21°
ΔMPFA = 21°

NSA = 131°   NSA =131°
MPFA = 90°
21°

© Springer-Verlag Berlin Heidelberg 2003

Fig. 2. Coxa vara with ΔNSA and ΔMPFA = 21°, therefore there is no greater trochanteric overgrowth. A valgus proximal femoral osteotomy will correct the upper femoral deformity. (*From* Paley D. Principles of deformity correction. 1st edition, 3rd printing. Berlin: Springer-Verlag; 2005; with permission.)

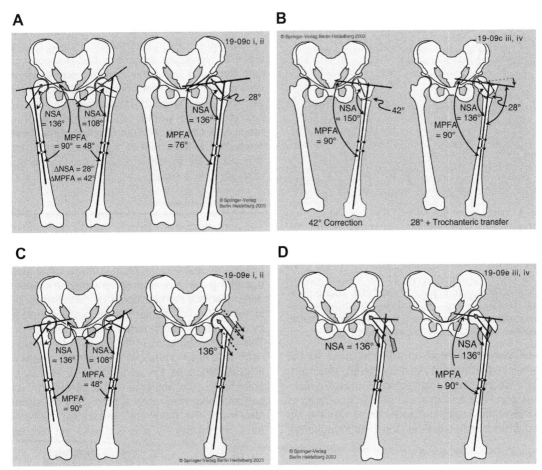

Fig. 3. (*A*) Coxa vara with ΔNSA = 28° and ΔMPFA = 42°, indicating that there is overgrowth of the greater trochanter together with coxa vara. If a valgus proximal femoral osteotomy is performed to correct the NSA, then the greater trochanter will still be too elevated. (*B*) If the valgus is increased to 42° to correct the MPFA to normal, then the NSA will be increased too much, to 150°. (*C*) To restore the NSA and the level of the greater trochanter, a Morscher osteotomy is performed removing a segment of greater trochanter and osteotomizing the femur at an angle of 130° to create a normal NSA. The trochanter is moved distal and lateral along this 130° slope. The congruity of the femoral head in the acetabulum does not change because the femoral head does not-adduct. (*D*) To restore the NSA and the level of the greater trochanter, a Wagner osteotomy is performed, increasing the angle of the proximal femur together with lateral-distal transfer of the greater trochanter. The congruity of the femoral head in the acetabulum changes because the femoral head adducts. (*From* Paley D. Principles of deformity correction. 1st edition, 3rd printing. Berlin: Springer-Verlag; 2005; with permission.)

INDICATIONS FOR PROXIMAL FEMORAL DEFORMITY SURGERY

There are 2 categories of surgery of the upper femur: intra-articular and extra-articular. Either or both may be indicated for joint preservation surgery of the hip. Indications for surgery are based on the history and physical, and the plain radiographic, computerized tomography, and magnetic resonance imaging studies. The presence of advanced arthrosis and stiffness may be a contraindication to joint preservation surgery. Even in asymptomatic patients there may be an indication for surgery because the prognosis for arthrosis and hip subluxation are known.

TYPES OF PROXIMAL FEMORAL DEFORMITIES

Extra-articular proximal femoral deformities that involve the entire proximal femur include varus, valgus, flexion, extension, internal and external rotation, and shortening. Extra-articular femoral deformities that involve parts of the proximal femur are deformities of the greater and lesser trochanter relative to the rest of the proximal femur (eg, overgrowth of the greater trochanter, lesser trochanter too proximal and medial compared with normal). The location of the greater and lesser trochanter is important because both trochanters serve as the insertion point of 2 critical muscle groups. If

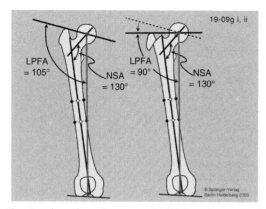

Fig. 4. When there is a normal NSA but the MPFA is increased, the greater trochanter is overgrown. This is the best indication for a greater trochanteric transfer without a proximal femoral osteotomy. With the Ganz relative neck lengthening osteotomy, the extra bone on the proximal aspect of the femoral neck is resected to prevent impingement. LPFA, lateral proximal femoral angle. (*From* Paley D. Principles of deformity correction. 1st edition, 3rd printing. Berlin: Springer-Verlag; 2005; with permission.)

the distance of these muscle insertions to the center of the femoral head is altered, lever arm dysfunction ensues manifested as muscle weakness and fatigue.[2] When the greater trochanter is too proximal, then the muscle tension on the hip abductors is reduced. When the greater trochanter

is too medial, as in cases of coxa breva, the abductor lever arm is reduced. The combination of reduced lever arm and reduced muscle tension leads to significant weakness that manifests as limp (lurch and Trendelenburg) and muscle fatigue during gait. If the lesser trochanter is too proximal and medial because of coxa breva, then the hip flexion may be weakened. Therefore, incorporating lateralization with distalization of the lesser trochanter is important to treat such weakness. It is important to test hip abduction and flexion strength before surgery.

Varus Osteotomy

The normal NSA of the femur is 130° ± 5°. Combined with a dysplastic acetabulum, valgus angles (>135°) predispose to subluxation. Although a pelvic osteotomy is the most important first step, combining it with a varus proximal femur osteotomy to stabilize the hip should be considered. The impact of the varus osteotomy is best exemplified by the Nishio varus osteotomy of the femur.[3] This varus osteotomy of the base of the femoral neck was used on its own to treat hip dysplasia (**Fig. 5**). Because the abductor lever arm is increased by this extreme varus osteotomy, the patient walks with minimal limp. This osteotomy challenges the belief that acetabular dysplasia must be treated by a pelvic, and not femoral,

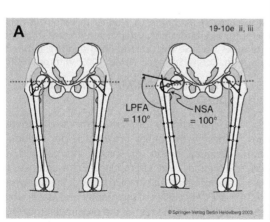

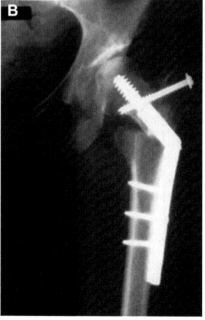

Fig. 5. (*A*) The Nishio osteotomy of the base of the neck. This osteotomy follows the intertrochanteric line posteriorly. It allows the proximal femur to be abducted to a greater degree because it does not elevate the greater trochanter as much. It lateralizes the greater trochanter, increasing the abductor lever arm. (*B*) Ten years after Nishio varus osteotomy. (*From* Paley D. Principles of deformity correction. 1st edition, 3rd printing. Berlin: Springer-Verlag; 2005; with permission.)

osteotomy,[3] and supports Bombelli's[1] concept that coxa vara applies medial forces on the acetabulum that can change its shape over time.

Because the center of rotation of angulation (CORA) of proximal femoral valgus is at the level of the base of the greater trochanter slightly proximal to a varus osteotomy, the osteotomy should be medially translated to avoid a secondary translation deformity.[2] For consideration of future hip replacement and to avoid secondary mechanical axis deviation at the knee, including the appropriate translation of the osteotomy is important to avoid creating a secondary translation deformity. An additional consideration with a varus osteotomy concerns the muscles attached to the 2 trochanters. Because varus osteotomy shortens the femur, it does not matter whether it is proximal or distal to the level of the lesser trochanter. Varus osteotomy has a greater effect on the greater trochanter. If the femur is in valgus and is brought to a normal 130° angle, then the tension (length) of the hip abductors is decreased but the lever arm is increased. The muscle tension can restore itself, whereas the lever arm cannot. This is therefore a net gain for the hip and reduces muscle fatigue and limp. If the NSA is at 130° and a varus osteotomy is performed, then the greater trochanter is elevated and loses both tension and lever arm, which can lead to a lurch or Trendelenburg gait. To avoid this, the greater trochanter should be transferred distally at the same time as the varus osteotomy, as was recommended by Müller (see **Fig. 2**).[4]

Valgus Osteotomy

Varus deformity of the proximal femur may be a sequela of previous treatment or a primary congenital deformity. The CORA for a varus deformity is very proximal in the femur and usually at the level of the center of the femoral head. Therefore an intertrochanteric or subtrochanteric valgus osteotomy needs to translate the distal segment laterally to avoid a secondary translation deformity. Coxa vara is often associated with other deformities, especially flexion and rotation. Correction of the proximal femoral deformity could combine correction in all 3 planes. The effect on the 2 trochanters needs to be considered. Because valgus osteotomy lengthens the femur, it moves the lesser trochanter distally if the osteotomy is proximal to the trochanter. This result may be desirable in cases of coxa breva in which the lesser trochanter is very proximal and medial, because the osteotomy will move it distally and laterally, improving its lever arm. The only danger is that, if there is already a flexion contracture, then this will aggravate the

situation. In most cases, I prefer to perform the osteotomy distal to the lesser trochanter to minimize the tension on the psoas tendon. The effect on the greater trochanter is to move it distally, increasing the tension on the hip abductors, and laterally, increasing the abductor lever arm. The increase of the abductor lever arm occurs until an optimal NSA of 130° is achieved. Angles greater than that begin to decrease the lever arm.

Proximal femoral osteotomy could be stabilized with internal or external fixation. Blade plate fixation is one of the best-designed methods for proximal femoral fixation because it offers excellent control of the osteotomy in the sagittal plane (**Fig. 6**). Sliding hip screws give excellent control and correction in the plane of fixation (plane of the neck of the femur) but less control in the sagittal plane. Locking plates for the proximal femur are a newer approach to fixate these osteotomies. Intramedullary fixation can be used for fixation if the deformity is first fixed and held corrected by an external fixator. This method, developed by Paley[2] and called fixator-assisted nailing, is best done with retrograde nailing. The external fixation pins are intentionally placed outside the path of the planned nail. The osteotomy is performed and the bone corrected to the desired position. The nail can then be introduced retrograde so as to spear the proximal segment in situ after the correction. Locking of the nail proximally and distally locks the correction into place.

Trochanteric Overgrowth

If trochanteric overgrowth is present, there are 3 approaches to correction of the proximal femoral anatomy: valgus intertrochanteric/subtrochanteric femoral osteotomy combined with lateral-distal transfer of greater trochanteric osteotomy (Wagner osteotomy) (see **Fig. 2**; **Fig. 7**)[5]; neck lengthening osteotomy of the intertrochanteric/trochanteric femur combined with lateral-distal transfer of greater trochanteric osteotomy (Morscher osteotomy) (see **Fig. 2**; **Fig. 8**)[6]; relative neck lengthening osteotomy (Ganz). Each of these has separate indications.

Valgus Intertrochanteric/Subtrochanteric Femoral Osteotomy Combined with Lateral-Distal Transfer of Greater Trochanteric Osteotomy (Wagner Osteotomy)

This type of osteotomy is used to change the part of the femoral head that is articulating with the acetabular dome (see **Figs. 2** and **7**).[5] The main indication is improved congruity, and reduction of joint forces when the femoral head is not spherical. The amount of rotation of the femoral head in

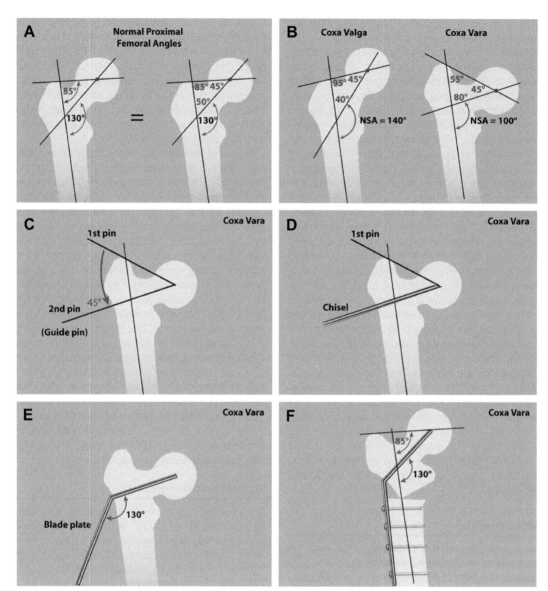

Fig. 6. (*A*) In the normal femur, the MPFA is 85°. The NSA is 130°. A triangle formed by the anatomic axis, the neck line, and the line from the greater trochanter to the center of the femoral head (proximal femur joint line) has an angle of 45° between the neck line and the proximal femoral joint line. (*B*) This 45° angle does not change with varus or valgus deformities and therefore can be used for planning of deformity correction of the upper femur. (*C*) For blade plate correction of a coxa vara deformity, insert a wire from the tip of the greater trochanter to the center of the femoral head, and another wire up the neck at 45° to the first wire. This procedure accurately places the neck line in the correct position relative to the joint line of the proximal femur. (*D*) The chisel is inserted in line with the second guidewire. (*E*) The chisel is replaced by the blade of the plate. (*F*) An osteotomy is made at the level of the base of the lesser trochanter. The amount of lateral translation is determined automatically by the distance to the plate because a plate with no offset is used. The rest of the fixation is added. For optimum mechanics, the length of the plate should be as long or longer than the length of the blade to neutralize the lever arms of fixation.

the acetabulum corresponds with the degree of re-orientation of the femoral neck out of varus. The other 2 osteotomies do not change the part of the femoral head that articulates with the dome of the acetabulum. The valgus, lateral translation

osteotomy reorients the femoral neck out of varus and lengthens the femur. The trochanteric transfer moves the tip of the greater trochanter to the level of the center of the femoral head distally and moves it laterally to increase the abductor moment

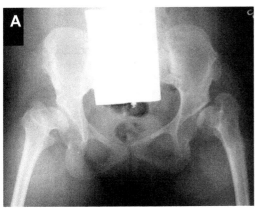
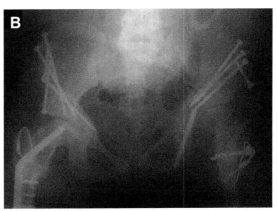

Fig. 7. (A) Bilateral severe hip dysplasia with an elliptical femoral head on the right side. (B) Wagner-type valgus osteotomy combined with distal lateral transfer of the greater trochanter combined with an extreme periacetabular osteotomy (PAO) osteotomy to gain coverage and congruity. The long axis of the elliptical femoral head is now horizontal (Bombelli principle).

arm. The combination of the two lengthens the femoral neck as well as the total length of the femur. Because valgus of the femoral neck moves it distally from the center of the hip joint, the lesser trochanter is advanced by this type of osteotomy. More advancement and lateralization can be achieved by performing the osteotomy proximal to the lesser trochanter. This osteotomy can be combined with derotation of the femur as well as sagittal correction.

Neck Lengthening Osteotomy of the Intertrochanteric/Subtrochanteric Femur Combined with Lateral-Distal Transfer of Greater Trochanteric Osteotomy (Morscher)

This type of osteotomy does not change the orientation of the femoral head in the acetabulum and therefore the congruity of the hip joint stays the same (see **Figs. 2** and **8**).[6] The indication for this is when there is no need to change the congruity of the joint. The NSA is created by the angle of the osteotomy. If a 130° NSA is desired then the intertrochanteric/subtrochanteric osteotomy is made at 130°. The greater trochanteric osteotomy is made at the same angle and shifted distally and laterally by sliding down this osteotomy line. The effect of the 2 osteotomies is to lengthen the femoral neck by lateralizing the greater trochanter and the femoral shaft, which also increases the total length of the femur. If the intertrochanteric osteotomy is performed proximal to the lesser trochanter, then the lesser trochanter can be moved laterally and distally. If it is made distal to the lesser trochanter, then there is no effect on the lesser trochanter.

Ganz Relative Neck Lengthening Osteotomy

This type of osteotomy is combined with a capsulotomy and hip dislocation (**Fig. 9**).[7] There is less danger to the circulation of the femoral head than with the other 2 greater trochanteric osteotomies because of the precautions taken to avoid injury to the vascular pedicle of the femoral head. A combined intra-articular and extra-articular impingement of the hip is best addressed with this osteotomy. Extra-articular impingement from the greater trochanter is better addressed with this method of trochanteric transfer than with the other methods, because all of the stable trochanter, which is the part of the greater trochanter that forms the lateral wall of the piriformis fossa, is resected. Also, the effect of the osteoplasty can be directly observed with this approach. This osteotomy creates a relative lengthening of the femoral neck on its superior/lateral surface because the trochanter is moved laterally and distally. The shaft of the femur is not lateralized, which is the major difference with the Morscher osteotomy. This difference may not be of any mechanical importance except for the insertion of the psoas tendon and the valgus effect that coxa breva has on the knee joint. The Ganz relative neck lengthening osteotomy does not lengthen the lower limb but the Morscher and Wagner do. It is important to understand the differences between these 3 osteotomies to choose the correct one for the correct indication. In addition, the relative neck lengthening and surgical dislocation can be combined with a Morscher or Wagner-type osteotomy of the intertrochanteric region.

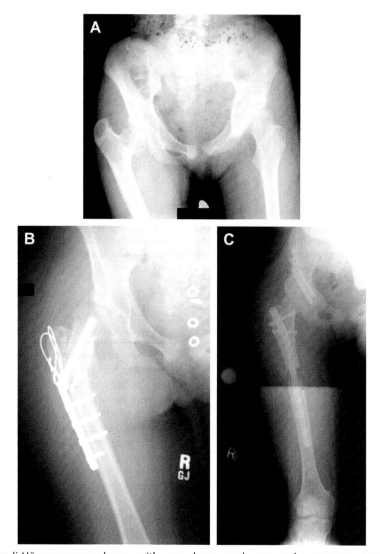

Fig. 8. (*A*) Conradi-Hünermann syndrome with coxa breva and vara and overgrown trochanter. There is a dysplastic acetabulum. (*B*) Treatment by Morscher osteotomy with neck lengthening and trochanteric and shaft lateral-distal transfer. The distal osteotomy was performed proximal to the lesser trochanter. The lesser trochanter was advanced distally and laterally. (*C*) A pelvic osteotomy was performed, followed 6 months later by a lengthening procedure for the short femur. The hip is well covered, which protects it from dislocation during the lengthening.

Intra-Articular Femoral Deformities

Deformities of the femoral head at its connection with the femoral neck are considered intra-articular. Deformities of the shape of the femoral head are intra-articular. Intra-capsular deformities of the femoral neck are also considered intra-articular. There are intra-articular and extra-articular surgical procedures for intra-articular deformities. For example, the deformity of the femoral head relative to the neck created by a slipped capital femoral epiphysis can be treated by an intra-articular reduction or osteotomy or an extra-articular reorientation osteotomy. The nonspherical femoral head can similarly be treated by a valgus intertrochanteric/subtrochanteric osteotomy or an intra-articular femoral head reduction osteotomy (FHRO) (**Figs. 10** and **11**).[8,9] Both of these solutions may still require a periacetabular osteotomy (PAO) for congruity and coverage because the aspherical femoral head would not be congruous if it was reoriented relative to the acetabulum. Performing the PAO allows the proximal

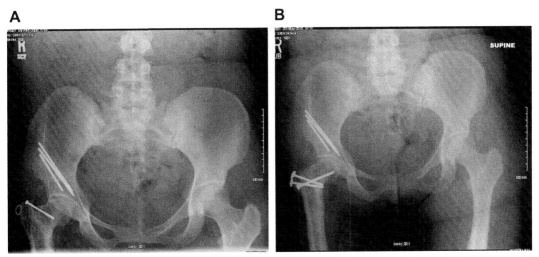

Fig. 9. (*A*) Congenital short femur with coxa vara and overgrown trochanter. A previous pelvic osteotomy had been performed. (*B*) Relative neck lengthening trochanteric transfer lateral to distal.

femur to be rendered valgus, combined with a similar amount of abduction of the acetabulum to maintain coverage and congruity.

THE ROLE OF CONTRACTURES AROUND THE HIP FOR HIP OSTEOTOMY

In the absence of an intra-articular bony obstruction caused by deformity of the femoral head, the limitations of corrective proximal femoral osteotomy are the surrounding soft tissues. The more extreme and the more chronic a hip deformity, the more likely there are to be associated contractures. For example, to correct a severe coxa vara, the femoral neck needs to be adducted by the degree of deformity.[2] The surrounding soft tissues may restrict this movement. For example, contractures of the lateral soft tissues around the hip may limit femoral neck adduction. The most common limiting soft tissue tether is the fascia lata and iliotibial band. The other tethers may include the hip abductors (gluteus medius and minimus), the tensor fascia lata, the gluteus maximus, and the hip joint capsule. Before embarking on a valgus osteotomy, it is important to perform a stress radiograph with the hip in maximum adduction. If the hip cannot be adducted by the amount of desired angular correction, then a valgus osteotomy cannot be performed without an accompanying soft tissue release. The easiest and most successful soft tissue release is surgical lengthening of the fascia lata at the musculo-tendinous junction with the tensor fascia lata and gluteus maximus muscles. This tissue can be transected at this level and the amount of adduction of the

hip reevaluated. If the hip adducts to the level required, then the valgus osteotomy can proceed. If not, then the condition is probably a contracture of the glutei. To address this requires a hip abductor slide procedure. In children, the apophysis can be split from anterior to two-thirds of the way posterior on the iliac crest, and the periosteum peeled distally with the glutei. This untethers the proximal femur and allows complete correction of even the most severe coxa vara deformities. After the proximal femur and pelvic osteotomy (if needed) are performed, the apophysis is pulled proximally and the level to which it reaches is marked with a pen. The iliac crest proximal to this mark is resected. The apophysis is closed after completion of this resection. The iliac crest can regenerate some of its height through the growth of this apophysis. The muscle tension of the glutei returns to normal. In adults, the proximal 1 cm of the crest is osteotomized and reflected distally with the attached glutei. After the osteotomies of the femur and, in some cases, pelvis, the iliac wing is shortened by the requisite amount to allow reattachment of the abductor muscles via the 1-cm top of the iliac crest. Both of these techniques are called abductor muscle slides and are only used in severe and chronic cases. The most common indication for this are the shepherd's crook deformity seen with fibrous dysplasia or congenital femoral deficiency. This technique forms part of the procedure described by Paley and Standard,[10] called the superhip procedure (**Fig. 12**).

Flexion contracture of the hip is another common, limiting factor. It can be addressed by

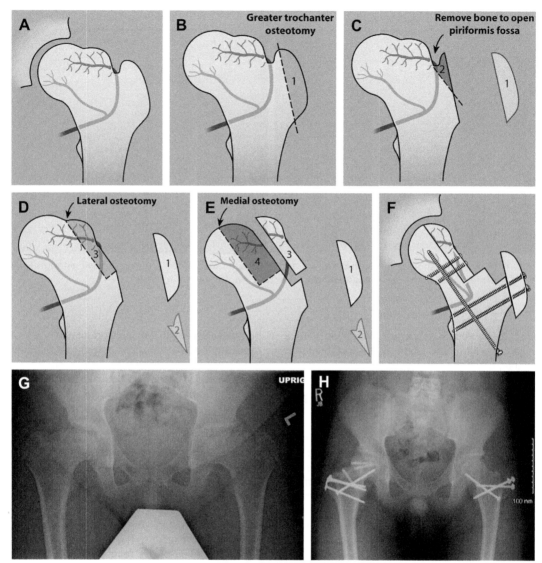

Fig. 10. (*A*) Coxa magna with deformity of femoral head. (*B*) Surgical dislocation performed with partial greater trochanter flip osteotomy. (*C*) Relative neck lengthening accomplished by removal of the stable trochanter, which forms the lateral wall of the piriformis fossa. (*D*) Osteotomy of the lateral part of the femoral head on its vascular pedicle while preserving the vascular supply of the medial femoral head. As an alternative, this segment could be resected to reduce the size of the femoral head (*H*, left hip). (*E*) Resection of central segment of femoral head while preserving the blood supply to the medial femoral head. (*F*) Reconstruction of the femoral head by reducing the lateral mobile head to the medial stable head. Fixation with headless screws and prophylactic neck screw to prevent fracture (*H*, right hip). The femoral head is now well contained. In some cases, this should be combined with a PAO. (*G*) Anteroposterior pelvis radiograph of bilateral coxa magna with elliptical femoral heads. There is impingement and the femoral head is uncovered. (*H*) Bilateral femoral head reduction osteotomies: right, performed by the Ganz FHRO method shown in *A–F*; left, performed by resecting the lateral part of the femoral head as in *D*.

lengthening of the psoas tendon as it passes over the pubis (fractional lengthening of the psoas). Release of the rectus femoris and the tensor fascia lata may also be needed. In the most severe cases, an abductor muscle slide is also used because most of the gluteus medius and minimus pass anterior to the center of rotation of the hip joint.

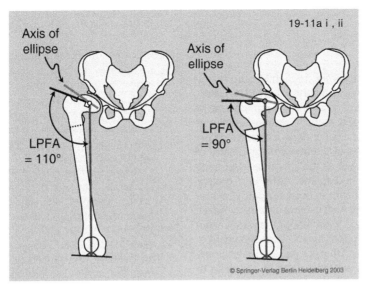

Fig. 11. For elliptical femoral heads, a valgus osteotomy to reorient the ellipse is one option (see also **Fig. 7**A, B). (*From* Paley D. Principles of deformity correction. 1st edition, 3rd printing. Berlin: Springer-Verlag; 2005; with permission.)

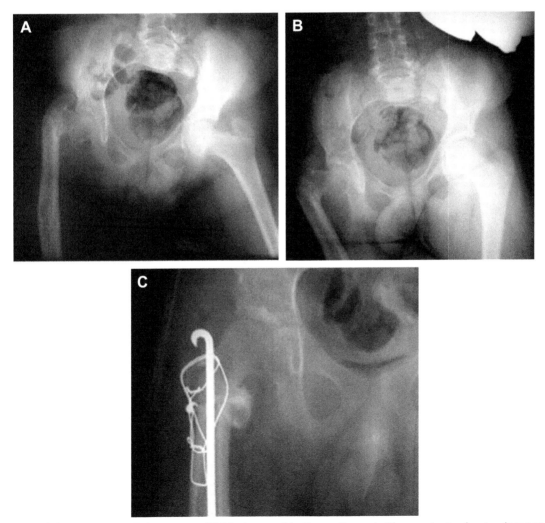

Fig. 12. (A) Severe congenital coxa vara. (B) Maximum adduction radiograph. The greater trochanter does not come down all of the way. (C) After superhip procedure with abductor muscle slide.

SUMMARY

Abnormalities of the femur frequently accompany acetabular dysplasia as primary or secondary deformities. Femoral surgery is often a component of surgical treatment of acetabular dysplasia either at the onset or to treat a secondary or residual deformity. Proper analysis of the abnormal geometry of the bony femur, as well as the abnormal lever arms around the hip related to the lesser and greater trochanteric positions, is an essential part of a successful surgical plan. An à la carte approach makes the most sense in the treatment of the wide variety of disorders of the upper femur. Over 100 years of hip surgery has proven that normalizing the anatomy and muscle forces around the hip to as close to normal as possible, extends the future life of the hip while also treating current pain and disability.

REFERENCES

1. Bombelli R. Structure and function in normal and abnormal hips: how to rescue mechanically jeopardized hips. 3rd edition. Berlin, Heidelberg, New York: Springer; 1993.
2. Paley D. Principles of deformity correction. 1st edition, 3rd printing. Berlin: Springer-Verlag; 2005.
3. Nishio A. Recent achievements in hip surgery. Fukuoka (Japan): Kyushu University; 1984.
4. Müller ME. Intertrochanteric osteotomy: indication, preoperative planning, technique. In: Schatzker J, editor. The intertrochanteric osteotomy. Berlin, Heidelberg, New York: Springer; 1984. p. 25–66.
5. Wagner H. Femoral osteotomies for congenital hip dislocation. In: Weil UH, editor. Progress in orthopedic surgery: acetabular dysplasia and skeletal dysplasia in childhood, vol. 2. Berlin, Heidelberg, New York: Springer; 1978. p. 85.
6. Hasler CC, Morscher EW. Femoral neck lengthening osteotomy after growth disturbance of the proximal femur. J Pediatr Orthop B 1999;8: 271–5.
7. Ganz R, Horowitz K, Leunig M. Treatment algorithm for combined femoral and periacetabular osteotomies in complex hip deformities. Clin Orthop Relat Res 2010;468(12):3168–80.
8. Paley D. The treatment of femoral head deformity and coxa magna by Ganz femoral head reduction osteotomy. Orthop Clin North Am 2011;42(3): 389–99.
9. Ganz R, Huff TW, Leunig M. Extended retinacular soft tissue flap for intra-articular hip surgery: surgical technique, indications, and results of its application. Instr Course Lect 2009;58:241–55.
10. Paley D, Standard SC. Treatment of congenital femoral deficiency. In: Wiesel S, editor. Operative techniques in orthopaedic surgery. Philadelphia: Lippincott Williams & Wilkins; 2010. p. 1202–23.

Imaging Hip Dysplasia in the Skeletally Mature

Cara Beth Lee, MD[a],*, Young-Jo Kim, MD, PhD[b,c]

KEYWORDS

- Hip dysplasia • Acetabular dysplasia • Hip preservation • Femoroacetabular impingement • FAI
- Hip radiographs • MRI hip • dGEMRIC

KEY POINTS

- When assessing a patient with hip pain, the recommended radiographs include: a well-centered anterior-posterior (AP) pelvis view, false profile images, and a 45 degree Dunn lateral view.
- The AP pelvis radiograph must be properly positioned to evaluate hip morphology: the sacrum should be centered over the symphysis and the distance from the symphysis to the sacrococcygeal joint should be 2 to 5 cm.
- Radiographic measures to diagnose acetabular dysplasia are: lateral and anterior center-edge angles less than 20 degrees and Tönnis roof angle greater than 10 degrees.
- Natural history studies suggest that patients with a lateral CE angle less than 16 degrees, Tönnis roof angle greater than 15 degrees, or femoral head subluxation, as demonstrated by a break in the Shenton line, are at high risk of developing osteoarthritis.
- Although the diagnoses of dysplasia and femoroacetabular impingement are established by radiographs, specialized imaging with magnetic resonance imaging (MRI) and computed tomography can guide treatment and surgical planning.
- Biochemical MR imaging modalities, such as T2 mapping, T1rho, and delayed gadolinium-enhanced MRI of cartilage (dGEMRIC), are evolving technologies that can detect early cartilage damage and enhance clinical decision-making in patients with established osteoarthritis.

BACKGROUND

Hip disease in adolescents and young adults presents as a spectrum of bony deformity that ranges from a shallow joint with symptomatic instability to an excessively constrained joint that may be painful as a result of femoroacetabular impingement (FAI). Acetabular dysplasia is characterized by an insufficient and, in some cases, steeply sloped acetabular roof that inadequately contains the femoral head. FAI occurs when an aspherical proximal femoral head-neck junction and/or an overly deep or improperly directed socket abut each other within a functional range of hip motion.

Acetabular dysplasia and FAI have both been associated with premature osteoarthritis (OA). In 1965, Murray[1] reviewed the radiographs of 200 patients with primary OA and found that more than 25% had features of acetabular dysplasia and 40% had a tilt deformity of the proximal femur. In 1975, Stulberg and colleagues[2] compared the radiographs of patients with idiopathic OA with

Funding sources disclosures: Dr Lee, none; Dr Kim, Orthopedic Research and Education Foundation, Siemens. Conflicts of interest: None.
a Center for Hip Preservation, Department of Orthopedics, Virginia Mason Medical Center, Lindeman Pavilion Level 6, 925 Seneca Street, Seattle, WA 98111, USA; b Department of Orthopedics, Harvard Medical School, Boston, MA, USA; c Adolescent and Young Adult Hip Program, Department of Orthopedics, Children's Hospital Boston, 300 Longwood Avenue, Hunnewell 221, Boston, MA 02115, USA
* Corresponding author.
E-mail address: cbleemd@gmail.com

orthopedic.theclinics.com

those of a cohort of patients who had been diagnosed with Perthes disease or slipped capital femoral epiphysis (SCFE) during childhood. They noted that 39% of the patients with OA had acetabular dysplasia and 40% had a pistol-grip femoral shape resembling the morphology of patients with SCFE and Perthes (**Fig. 1**). Current understanding of the pathomechanics of FAI invites reinterpretation of hips with tilt and pistol-grip deformities to be categorized as cam-type impingement lesions. With this perspective, Clohisy and colleagues[3] conducted a multicenter review of patients less than 50 years of age who had undergone total hip replacement between 1975 and 2005. Of 337 hip replacements performed for OA, radiographs showed acetabular dysplasia in 48% and impingement (including post-SCFE) lesions in 42%. Thus, 90% of patients with OA that led to hip replacement before age 50 years in this study had identifiable, predisposing bony deformities. Hip-preserving surgical procedures, such as periacetabular osteotomy (PAO), surgical hip dislocation, and hip arthroscopy, offer safe and effective options to correct these abnormalities. Mid-term to long-term follow-up of these procedures indicate that success is largely determined by the degree of cartilage damage at the time of surgery.[4–13] Thus, it is important to understand the varieties of hip disorders and identify

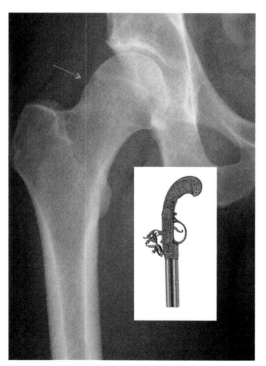

Fig. 1. Pistol-grip deformity. There is diminished offset of the femoral head-neck junction (*arrow*).

mechanically compromised hips in a timely manner. Imaging plays a central role in detecting and diagnosing the anatomic deformity. In addition, imaging measures are increasingly used to stage the degree of deformity and joint degeneration to guide prognosis and assess the impact of hip-preserving procedures, such as PAO and osteochondroplasty for FAI.

Acetabular Dysplasia

Acetabular dysplasia is characterized by a deficient acetabular weight-bearing zone that overloads the articular cartilage and labrum and can lead to OA. It predominantly affects women and may be a sequela of developmental dysplasia of the hip (DDH), or it may present in an adolescent or adult with no history of childhood hip disease. The severity of dysplasia ranges from a subluxated or dislocated hip to more subtle variants of a mildly shallow acetabulum that may go unrecognized until symptoms develop. Patients typically present with insidious onset of activity-related groin or lateral hip pain.[14] Most have a positive impingement sign (pain with combined hip flexion, adduction, and internal rotation); many have a limp and positive Trendelenburg sign.[14] Acetabular dysplasia is most commonly identified as deficient lateral femoral head coverage, but it may also involve significant anterior deficiency, which is identified on a false-profile view.[15] Acetabular dysplasia is frequently associated with proximal femoral deformities, such as coxa valga, femoral anteversion, and femoral head abnormalities. With growing awareness of FAI, it is now recognized that many patients with acetabular dysplasia also have FAI morphology of decreased femoral head-neck offset.[16] Among the hip deformities that lead to OA, the natural history of acetabular dysplasia is best understood. In 1939, Wiberg[17] published an extensive review of hip dysplasia and was the first to quantify acetabular coverage by describing the center-edge (CE) angle. He defined a CE angle less than 20° as abnormal and noted a linear relationship with lower coverage angles and subluxation corresponding with earlier development of OA. In a series of 286 patients, Murphy and colleagues[18] reported that no patient with a CE angle less than 16° and acetabular roof index greater than 15° reached age 65 years with a well-functioning hip.

FAI

In 1935, Smith-Petersen[19] first described pathologic impingement between the acetabular rim and proximal femur in a case series of patients whose disorders included protrusio acetabuli, previous SCFE, and OA. He recommended acetabuloplasty, even for patients with predominantly femoral-sided lesions, because of concern about weakening the femoral neck with excessive resection. Although the association between proximal femoral deformity and OA was repeatedly observed in subsequent decades,[1,2,20] it was not until Ganz and colleagues[21] introduced the surgical dislocation in the early 1990s that operative access to manage FAI became feasible.

On the femoral side, the pathologic morphology involves a prominent or aspherical femoral head-neck junction. With flexion and internal rotation of the hip, the incongruent articulation between the femoral head-neck junction and the acetabulum results in a cam-type impingement that can cause acetabular chondral delamination and labral damage.[22–24] Patients with normal femoral head-neck shape but increased femoral retroversion may impinge because of the limited capacity for combined flexion and internal rotation.

On the acetabular side, overcoverage can restrict motion because of pincer-type impingement.[22] The excess coverage may be global and severe, such as in protrusio acetabuli, mild, as in coxa profunda, or focally anterior, as occurs in acetabular retroversion. Most cases of protrusio are idiopathic, although it is associated with other conditions, such as Marfan disease and rheumatoid arthritis.[25–27] With pincer impingement, the femoral neck impacts the deep anterior acetabular rim in flexion, which causes outside-in labral damage.[22] Often, there may be combined cam and pincer impingement. Patients with FAI present with insidious onset of activity-related groin pain and positive impingement test on physical examination.[28]

There may be overlap in hips with dysplasia and impingement morphology. Acetabular retroversion has been reported to occur with acetabular dysplasia in a range from 17% to 38%[29–31]; the incidence of insufficient femoral head-neck offset with acetabular dysplasia is more than 70%.[16]

IMAGING
Anteroposterior View

Plain film imaging to screen for hip abnormalities begins with an anteroposterior (AP) pelvis radiograph. For a supine film, both hips are internally rotated 15° to neutralize femoral anteversion, which gives a true AP image of the proximal femur in most patients. The x-ray beam is centered at the midpoint between the superior border of the pubic symphysis and a horizontal line connecting the anterior superior iliac spines with a tube-to-film distance of 120 cm. Quantitative measures vary with the position of the pelvis; therefore, the first step in evaluating an AP pelvis radiograph is to determine whether it is

appropriately positioned with respect to tilt and rotation.[32] To determine proper rotation around the longitudinal axis, the center of the sacrum and coccyx should be in line with the pubic symphysis and the ilia, obturator foramina and acetabular teardrops symmetric. Siebenrock and colleagues[33] determined that the distance from the top of the pubic symphysis to the sacrococcygeal (SC) joint averages 32 mm in men and 47 mm in women. Distances of 2 to 5 cm from the top of the symphysis to the SC joint are considered acceptable for radiographic positioning of tilt. The SC joint can sometimes be obscure, so others have accepted a distance of 0 to 2 cm from the symphysis to the tip of the coccyx.[29]

The supine AP image is helpful for qualitative assessment of OA and femoral head shape, as well as qualitative and quantitative measures of acetabular coverage and orientation. Pelvic tilt, the forward (flexion or inclination) or backward (extension or reclination) rotation of the pelvis around the transverse axis, varies by individual and position. The pelvis extends with movement from supine to standing, which alters acetabular and joint space measures.[34] Because of this variation in tilt, some investigators recommend standing AP pelvis radiographs to evaluate functional joint space width and to quantify acetabular parameters in dysplasia.[35]

When reviewing the AP pelvis radiograph, it is helpful to develop a systematic routine to screen for acetabular and femoral abnormalities. The following are commonly used measures of acetabular morphology:

1. Lateral CE angle. This angle is formed by the intersection of a line from the center of the femoral head to the lateral rim of the acetabulum and a second line that is perpendicular to a line connecting the center of the femoral heads (**Fig. 2**).[17] Wiberg[17] defined a CE angle greater than 25° as normal and less than 20° as dysplastic. The upper limit of normal has not been clearly defined; however, CE angle greater than 40° indicates a deep acetabulum that may be at risk for pincer impingement (**Figs. 3** and **4**).
2. Acetabular roof angle, or Tönnis angle.[36] This angle is determined by a line between the femoral head centers (or parallel to it) and a second line that connects the most medial and lateral margins of the sclerotic acetabular weight-bearing zone, or the sourcil (the original description used a line perpendicular to the vertical axis of the sacrum to represent the transverse pelvic axis but, in our experience, this axis is more accurately denoted by a line connecting the centers of the femoral heads).

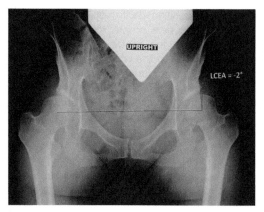

Fig. 2. Lateral CE angle. This angle is determined by the intersection of a line from the center of the femoral head to the lateral rim of the acetabulum and a second line that is perpendicular to a line connecting the center of the femoral heads. Normal lateral CE angle is 25° to 35°.

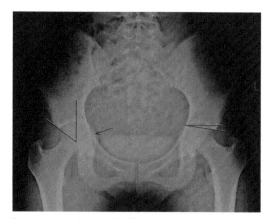

Fig. 4. Protrusio acetabuli. In this patient, the lateral CE angle is greater than 40°, the Tönnis angle is negative, and the femoral head is medial to the ilioischial line. In addition, this example shows the teardrop medial to the iliopectineal line (*arrow*), another indicator of protrusio.

Normal acetabular roof angles range between 0° and 10°. Dysplastic hips have a steeper roof, with Tönnis angles greater than 10° (**Fig. 5**), whereas overcoverage is characterized by a downsloping or negative roof angle (see **Figs. 3** and **4**).

3. Shenton line. This line describes the curve from the top of the obturator foramen to the medial, inferior femoral neck.[37] In a normal hip, this arc maintains a smooth contour. Disruption of the Shenton line greater than 5 mm indicates dysplasia with femoral head subluxation (**Fig. 6**).

4. Cross-over sign. The anterior acetabular wall is a continuation of the superior public ramus and is more horizontally oriented. The posterior wall extends from the lateral ischium and is more

vertical. In a normal hip, the anterior and posterior acetabular walls meet at the lateral rim on an AP radiograph. The cross-over sign is an indicator of acetabular retroversion or focal anterior overcoverage; it is positive if the anterior acetabular wall projects lateral to the posterior wall (**Fig. 7**).[38] This measure may be falsely positive with increased pelvic inclination.

5. Posterior wall sign. The rim of the posterior wall of the acetabulum should be in line with or lateral to the center of the femoral head on an AP radiograph. The posterior wall sign is positive if the rim is medial to the center of the head, which denotes insufficient posterior coverage and occurs with acetabular retroversion or global acetabular dysplasia (see **Fig. 7**).[38]

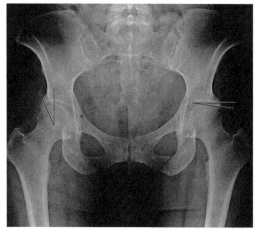

Fig. 3. Coxa profunda. In this patient, the lateral CE angle is high, the Tönnis angle is negative, and the acetabular teardrop is medial to the ilioischial line (*arrow*).

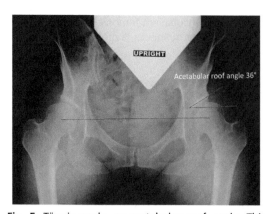

Fig. 5. Tönnis angle, or acetabular roof angle. This angle is the intersection of a line connecting the center of the femoral heads with a line parallel to the sourcil of the acetabulum. Normal Tönnis angle is 0° to 10°.

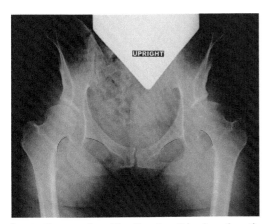

Fig. 6. Shenton line. The Shenton line describes the arc from the inferior femoral neck to the superior obturator foramen, which should form a smooth contour. In this example of a patient with bilateral acetabular dysplasia, there is disruption of the Shenton line on the left hip.

6. Ischial spine sign. This sign strongly correlates with the cross-over sign as another indicator of acetabular retroversion, but it is less affected by pelvic tilt.[39] It is considered positive if the ischial spine projects medial to the iliopectineal line (see **Fig. 7**).[40]
7. Ilioischial line. The floor of the acetabular fossa, which corresponds radiographically with the acetabular teardrop, and the position of the femoral head should be examined relative to

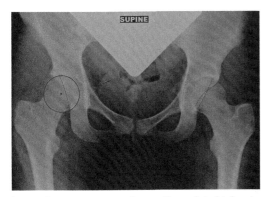

Fig. 7. Cross-over, posterior wall, and ischial spine signs. The anterior (*dotted line*) and posterior walls (*solid lines*) should meet at the lateral rim of acetabulum on the AP view. The cross-over sign is an indication of acetabular retroversion and is considered positive when the anterior wall is lateral to the posterior wall. The ischial spine sign is also associated with acetabular retroversion and is positive if the ischial spine projects medially to the iliopectineal line (*arrows*). The posterior wall sign is positive if the rim of the wall is medial to the center of the head, which indicates insufficient posterior coverage.

the ilioischial line as additional measures of acetabular depth in patients with a high lateral CE angle or negative roof angle. In coxa profunda, the teardrop touches or is medial to the ilioischial line (see **Fig. 3**).[41] The teardrop can be medial to the ilioischial line in dysplastic hips; therefore, this radiographic sign must be interpreted in context. In protrusio acetabuli, the femoral head is medial to this line (see **Fig. 4**).

False-Profile View

The false-profile view is a lateral image of the acetabulum tangential to the anterior acetabular rim that allows measurement of anterior femoral head coverage.[15] It is sensitive to detect mild dysplasia or early joint space narrowing that may not be evident on the AP view.[42] The image is obtained standing with the affected hip positioned against the cassette and the ipsilateral foot parallel to it. The pelvis is rotated 65° away from the cassette and the x-ray beam is centered on the femoral head with a tube-to-film distance of 90 cm. The anterior center-edge angle is determined by a vertical line through the center of the femoral head and a second line from the center of the head to the edge of the sclerotic weight-bearing zone of the anterior acetabulum. Similar to the lateral CE angle, normal values are 25° to 35°, with less than 20° considered dysplastic, and greater than 40° indicating overcoverage (**Fig. 8**).

Abduction-Internal Rotation (von Rosen) View

Although initially described for the evaluation of DDH in children, the von Rosen view[43] is a functional radiograph that is useful for preoperative planning, as well as a screening tool to identify patients with incongruence or advanced OA who may fare poorly with joint-preserving procedures.[44] The image is obtained with both legs in maximal abduction and internal rotation, which reflects the joint congruence that can be achieved with rotation of the acetabular fragment from a periacetabular osteotomy (**Fig. 9**).

Lateral Views

Lateral views of the hip are useful for visualizing proximal femoral morphology. The most commonly used lateral radiographs are the cross-table lateral and the frog-leg lateral. The cross-table view is obtained with the patient supine and the uninvolved hip and knee flexed greater than 80°. The x-ray beam is directed parallel to the table at a 45° angle to the symptomatic hip and centered on the femoral head. The affected hip is internally rotated 15° to target the beam tangential to the anterosuperior head-neck junction.[45] The frog-leg lateral view is

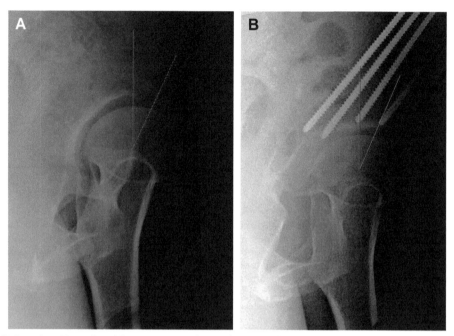

Fig. 8. (*A*) Anterior CE angle. This measure is obtained on the false-profile view and is the angle between a vertical line through the center of the femoral head and a second line from the center of the head to the sclerotic anterior edge of the acetabular sourcil. In this example, the anterior CE angle is 0°. The dashed line indicates where the sourcil should extend to achieve normal coverage, which corresponds with an angle of 25°. (*B*) The same patient after periacetabular osteotomy with improved anterior coverage as noted by a normal anterior CE angle (*red lines*).

obtained with the patient supine; the affected hip is abducted 45° with the knee flexed 30° to 40° and the heel resting against the medial side of the contralateral knee.[46] The beam is directed at a point midway between the anterior superior iliac spine and the pubic symphysis with a tube-to-cassette distance of 90 cm.

The α angle is widely used to quantify the femoral head-neck junction.[47] It was originally described from oblique axial magnetic resonance (MR) images but is now commonly measured on

lateral radiographs. The angle is formed by the intersection of a line along the axis of the center of the femoral neck passing through the center of the femoral head and a second line from the center of the femoral head to the point on the femoral head-neck junction where the head ceases to be spherical (**Fig. 10**). In the initial study, the mean α angle was 42° (range 33°–48°) in the control group and 74° (range 55°–95°) in the group with symptomatic impingement. In general, an α angle of 55° or more is considered abnormal when

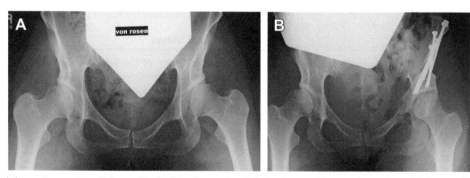

Fig. 9. (*A*) von Rosen view. Taken with the hips in maximal abduction and internal rotation, this image shows the congruence that can be expected between the weight-bearing acetabulum and the femoral head when planning periacetabular osteotomy. (*B*) Postoperative AP view of the same patient.

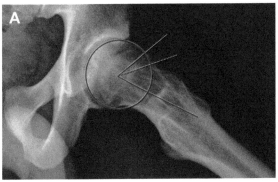 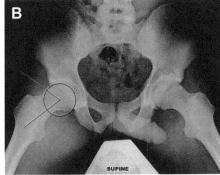

Fig. 10. (A) α Angle, frog-leg lateral view. The α angle is formed by a line along the center of the femoral neck passing through the center of the femoral head and a second line from the center of the femoral head to the point where the head-neck junction becomes aspherical. This example is a cam lesion with α angle greater than 55°. The dotted line depicts the threshold for normal, which is less than 50°. (B) α Angle, 45° Dunn-Rippstein lateral view. This radiograph view shows the superolateral femoral head-neck region, which is the most common location of diminished offset. In this example of a patient with bilateral cam lesions, the femoral head is posteriorly translated relative to the center of the femoral neck. Thus, the α angle is drawn with a line parallel to the center of the femoral neck that intersects the center of the femoral head. If it were drawn through the center of the femoral neck, it would be anterior to the center of the femoral head, which is frequently the case in patients with prior SCFE.

supported by other clinical findings of FAI. In a retrospective comparison, the frog-leg lateral view was found to be more accurate than AP and cross-table lateral images for assessing femoral head-neck offset and α angle.[46] Meyer and colleagues[48] examined 6 radiographic views (not including the frog-leg lateral) and determined that the 45° Dunn-Rippstein lateral (45 degree Dunn) view was the most sensitive for assessing the α angle (see **Fig. 10**B). A recent report noted 96% sensitivity to detect a cam lesion with a Dunn view compared with 71% on a cross-table lateral image using radial magnetic resonance imaging (MRI) as the standard.[49] The 45 degree Dunn view is obtained with the patient supine and the affected hip in 45° flexion, 20° abduction, and neutral rotation. The beam direction and distance are identical to the frog-leg lateral radiograph.

Tables 1 and **2** summarize normal and pathologic measures on plain radiographs.

Computed Tomography

Computed tomography (CT) scans can be reformatted in multiple planes to provide a more accurate and comprehensive rendering of bony structure compared with two-dimensional radiography. CT has added a great deal to the knowledge of normal and dysplastic acetabular anatomy. Several investigations have delineated acetabular version in asymptomatic populations and consistently show that acetabular anteversion is greater in women than men,[50,51] a finding that

corresponds with measures obtained from osteological collections of human skeletons.[52] Anda and colleagues[53] described the acetabular sector angles, which divide the acetabulum into anterior

Table 1 Acetabular measures on plain radiographs		
	AP Image	**False-Profile Image**
Normal	LCEA 25°–35° TA 0°–10°	ACEA 25°–35°
Acetabular dysplasia	LCEA <20° TA >10°	ACEA <20°
Coxa profunda	Teardrop medial to ilioischial line LCEA >40° TA <0°	ACEA >40°
Protrusio acetabuli	Femoral head medial to ilioischial line LCEA 40° TA <0°	ACEA >40°
Acetabular retroversion	Cross-over sign Ischial spine sign	—

Note: CE angles from 20° to 25° and 35° to 40° are considered borderline normal.

Abbreviations: ACEA, anterior CE angle; LCEA, lateral CE angle; TA, Tönnis angle.

Table 2
Proximal femoral measures on plain radiographs

	AP Image	45° Dunn Lateral View
Normal	Spherical head-neck junction	α Angle <50°
Cam lesion	Aspherical head-neck junction Pistol-grip deformity	α Angle >55°

Note: α angles between 50° and 55° are considered borderline normal.

and posterior sections, to define more accurately global acetabular coverage (**Fig. 11**). Although anteversion and sector angles are generally measured at the center of the femoral head,[54] anteversion increases from cephalad to caudad in the normal hip and has wide variability in dysplastic hips.[55] In a CT investigation of acetabular retroversion, Perreira and colleagues[56] concluded that retroversion is not caused by isolated posterior insufficiency or anterior overcoverage but reflects torsion of the acetabulum and ischial spine segment. More recent investigations suggest that it is more accurate to define the acetabular opening based on measures of an acetabular rim plane, rather than from a single axial slice.[57]

Klaue and colleagues[58] described a CT method to determine femoral head coverage to simulate correction and aid surgical planning of both pelvic and femoral osteotomies. Using a three-dimensional (3D) graphics program, their technique creates a topographic map of the acetabulum and femoral head by outlining overlapping contours on sequential axial images. CT-derived surface contour maps to define femoral head coverage have shown that the deficiency in

dysplasia is global, rather than isolated to the anterolateral acetabulum as had previously been thought.[59] Janzen and colleagues[60] described a technique to measure femoral head coverage by reformatting vertical planar images from 3D CT to create CE angles in 10° increments circumferentially around the acetabular rim. This method was subsequently used to compare graphically the coverage before and after periacetabular osteotomy.[61] Ito and colleagues[62] reported good correlation between 3D CT and conventional radiographic measures for CE angle and Tönnis roof angles; however, they recommended the detailed evaluation of 3D CT to individualize surgical planning because of the wide variability in the location and degrees of deficiency in patients with acetabular dysplasia.

CT is a powerful tool to assess bony anatomy. Understanding of the variability in normal and dysplastic pelvic morphology is important when planning reorientation procedures of the acetabulum, as well as implant positioning in arthroplasty. However, each of the studies discussed earlier used graphics programs to manipulate CT image data after reformatting, which is time consuming and rarely available in the clinical setting. Moreover, CT scans can be subject to error. As previously discussed, pelvic inclination changes from supine to standing, but current CT imaging can only be performed with a patient supine. Pelvic obliquity and tilt are determined by the patient's position in the gantry, which can affect acetabular measures.[63] 3D reformatting is required to correct positioning and improve accuracy but is not routinely performed with standard CT imaging.[64,65] Apart from these concerns, the primary limit to widespread use of CT imaging for acetabular dysplasia is the increasing worry about radiation exposure,[66] particularly in this population of young, female patients in whom radiation-associated cancer risks are highest.[67]

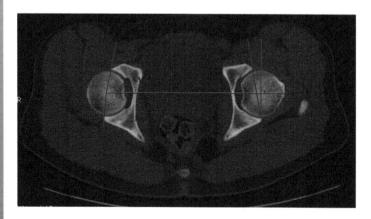

Fig. 11. Axial CT measurement of acetabular anteversion and sector angles. The anterior (AASA) and posterior acetabular sector angles (PASA) are determined by a line connecting the center of the femoral heads and a line to the anterior and posterior acetabular rims, respectively. Acetabular anteversion (AA) is the angle formed between a line perpendicular to the line from the center of the femoral heads and a line contacting the anterior and posterior rim.

MRI

Similar to CT, MR images can be reformatted in multiple planes to provide a thorough analysis of the 3D anatomy of the hip and pelvis. In addition to comprehensive assessment of bony disorders, MRI provides superior detail of cartilage, labrum, synovium, and soft tissues.[68] Clinically relevant labral tears are infrequent in the absence of a bony anomaly, such as a proximal femoral cam lesion.[69] MRI radial views can simultaneously detect labral disorders[70,71] and subtle abnormalities of the femoral head-neck junction that may be missed on radiographs (**Fig. 12**).[72,73] Acetabular and femoral version can be measured with axial views through the roof of the acetabulum and the femoral neck and condyles, respectively.

Because of the spherical shape of the articular surfaces and thin cartilage, MRI in the hip remains complex and requires high resolution and contrast/noise ratio to differentiate bone, cartilage, capsule, and labrum.[74] MR arthrography is the gold standard for identifying labral disorders[75–77] but has a higher false-positive rate than noncontrast MRI.[78] Techniques using small pixel size[79] and higher field resolution[80] are improving the accuracy to detect labral and cartilage disorders without the need for contrast, but sensitivity to distinguish acetabular chondral delamination is still lacking.[74,81,82]

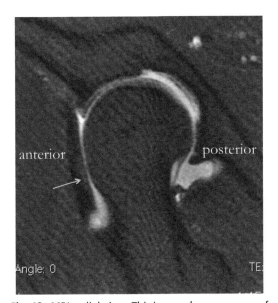

Fig. 12. MRI radial view. This image shows an area of diminished femoral head-neck offset (*arrow*) in a patient in whom AP and cross-table lateral radiographs were normal.

Biochemical MRI

Biochemical MRI reflects the structure and molecular composition of cartilage. These evolving techniques have improved the ability to detect degenerative changes not appreciable on plain MRI. Currently, the primary modalities are T2 mapping, T1rho, and delayed gadolinium-enhanced MRI of cartilage (dGEMRIC).

Normal articular cartilage is composed of 3 layers: a superficial layer with collagen fibers arranged parallel to the cartilage surface, high collagen and water content, and low proteoglycan concentration; a middle zone with obliquely oriented collagen fibers, high proteoglycan content, and lower collagen and water volumes than the superficial layer; and a deep zone with densely packed collagen fibers oriented perpendicular to the articular surface, the highest proteoglycan content, and lowest water concentration.[83]

T2 relaxation times are sensitive to the interaction between collagen and water molecules and can be mapped to show the layered architecture of cartilage.[84] In normal cartilage, T2 mapping reveals a zonal gradation with low signal intensity in the deep layer that increases in the intermediate and superficial layers. T2 signal increases with disruption of this highly organized structure and the increased water content that occurs with cartilage degeneration.[85,86] Interpretation of T2 results can be complicated by competing tissue factors[87] and structural responses to loading.[88,89] T2* mapping has shorter acquisition time and the capacity for 3D imaging; however, it is more susceptible to artifacts at the bone-cartilage interface and from foreign body particles.[90]

One of the first events in cartilage degeneration is loss of proteoglycan content,[91] which is not detected on T2 images.[92] Thus, T2 mapping is not sensitive to early stages of OA. T1rho is a technique that is responsive to changes in the collagen structure and water content, as well as proteoglycan concentration.[93] However, similar to T2, because T1rho is influenced by alterations in various components, the competing effects make accurate interpretation of T1rho values difficult and prone to error.[87]

Of the available biochemical MRI modalities, dGEMRIC has been most widely studied in clinical settings, particularly the hip. This method takes advantage of the highly negatively charged glycosaminoglycan (GAG) molecules that comprise the proteoglycan component of cartilage. With loss of proteoglycan in early OA, there is a decrease in charge density that can be measured by a mobile ion probe, such as gadolinium pentetate (Gd-DTPA^{2-}).[94] The technique

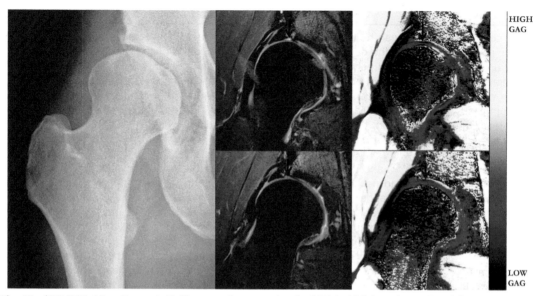

HIGH
GAG

LOW
GAG

Fig. 13. dGEMRIC. AP radiograph (*left*), coronal proton density MRI (*middle*), and associated dGEMRIC images (*right*) of a patient with symptomatic dysplasia. The color scale reflects the T1 relaxation time, which is proportional to the GAG content of the cartilage. Normal cartilage with a high concentration of GAG is yellow. This patient has moderate-to-low dGEMRIC measures. Blue arrows highlight the zone of lowest GAG concentration in the cartilage of the lateral acetabulum.

involves injection of intravenous contrast material and then MRI imaging after a delay of 30 minutes to allow time for contrast penetration into the articular cartilage.[95,96] This method yields an indirect arthrogram in addition to enhancement of articular cartilage that can be quantitatively measured for GAG content after T1 mapping (**Fig. 13**). Kim and colleagues[97] found that dGEMRIC measures correlate with pain and the severity of acetabular dysplasia and may be an early indicator of OA in this population. Subsequent work showed that the dGEMRIC index was the most important predictor of early outcome after periacetabular osteotomy compared with standard MRI, radiographs, and clinical measures.[98] This modality is sensitive to early cartilage deterioration and has been used to delineate patterns of articular damage in FAI,[99,100] Perthes disease,[101] and SCFE.[102] Both hips can be imaged with one intravenous contrast injection, which is beneficial in disease entities that are often bilateral, such as dysplasia and FAI. The primary drawback of dGEMRIC is the risk associated with gadolinium injection, which requires caution in patients with renal impairment.

SUMMARY

Hip disorders in the young adult manifest along a continuum that ranges from an excessively constrained, impinging joint, to an overly shallow, unstable hip. Knowledge of simple measures on plain radiographs can aid in efficient and accurate

identification of mechanically compromised hips that may be at risk for premature OA. Improvements in joint-preserving surgery have shown promise in delaying or preventing progression of articular degeneration; thus, timely diagnosis is important. Once a diagnosis is established, specialized imaging can be individualized to supplement surgical planning, assess the degree of cartilage damage, and facilitate discussion regarding the prognosis of hip-preserving procedures.

REFERENCES

1. Murray RO. The aetiology of primary osteoarthritis of the hip. Br J Radiol 1965;38:810–24.
2. Stulberg SC, Cordell LD, Harris WH, et al. Unrecognized childhood hip disease: a major cause of idiopathic osteoarthritis of the hip. In: Ramsey PL, MacEwen GD, editors. The hip, proceedings of the third open scientific meeting of the Hip Society. St Louis (MO): CV Mosby; 1975. p. 212–8.
3. Clohisy JC, Dobson MA, Robison JF, et al. Radiographic structural abnormalities associated with premature, natural hip-joint failure. J Bone Joint Surg Am 2011;93(Suppl 2):3–9.
4. Clohisy JC, Schutz AL, St John L, et al. Periacetabular osteotomy: a systematic literature review. Clin Orthop Relat Res 2009;467:2041–52.
5. Ganz R, Klaue K, Vinh TS, et al. A new periacetabular osteotomy for the treatment of hip dysplasias: technique and preliminary results. 1988. Clin Orthop Relat Res 2004;(418):3–8.

6. Matheney T, Kim YJ, Zurakowski D, et al. Intermediate to long-term results following the Bernese periacetabular osteotomy and predictors of clinical outcome. J Bone Joint Surg Am 2009;91:2113–23.

7. Millis MB, Kain M, Sierra R, et al. Periacetabular osteotomy for acetabular dysplasia in patients older than 40 years: a preliminary study. Clin Orthop Relat Res 2009;467:2228–34.

8. Steppacher SD, Tannast M, Ganz R, et al. Mean 20-year followup of Bernese periacetabular osteotomy. Clin Orthop Relat Res 2008;466:1633–44.

9. Beck M, Leunig M, Parvizi J, et al. Anterior femoroacetabular impingement: part II. Midterm results of surgical treatment. Clin Orthop Relat Res 2004;(418):67–73.

10. Botser IB, Smith TW Jr, Nasser R, et al. Open surgical dislocation versus arthroscopy for femoroacetabular impingement: a comparison of clinical outcomes. Arthroscopy 2011;27:270–8.

11. Clohisy JC, St John LC, Schutz AL. Surgical treatment of femoroacetabular impingement: a systematic review of the literature. Clin Orthop Relat Res 2010;468:555–64.

12. Larson CM, Giveans MR. Arthroscopic management of femoroacetabular impingement: early outcomes measures. Arthroscopy 2008;24:540–6.

13. Matsuda DK, Carlisle JC, Arthurs SC, et al. Comparative systematic review of the open dislocation, mini-open, and arthroscopic surgeries for femoroacetabular impingement. Arthroscopy 2011;27:252–69.

14. Nunley RM, Prather H, Hunt D, et al. Clinical presentation of symptomatic acetabular dysplasia in skeletally mature patients. J Bone Joint Surg Am 2011;93(Suppl 2):17–21.

15. Lequesne M, de Sèze S. False profile of the pelvis. A new radiographic incidence for the study of the hip. Its use in dysplasias and different coxopathies. Rev Rhum Mal Osteoartic 1961;28:643–52 [in French].

16. Clohisy JC, Nunley RM, Carlisle JC, et al. Incidence and characteristics of femoral deformities in the dysplastic hip. Clin Orthop Relat Res 2009;467:128–34.

17. Wiberg G. Studies on dysplastic acetabula and congenital subluxation of the hip joint. Acta Chir Scand 1939;83(Suppl 58):5–135.

18. Murphy SB, Ganz R, Muller ME. The prognosis in untreated dysplasia of the hip. A study of radiographic factors that predict the outcome. J Bone Joint Surg Am 1995;77:985–9.

19. Smith-Petersen MN. The classic: treatment of malum coxae senilis, old slipped upper femoral epiphysis, intrapelvic protrusion of the acetabulum, and coxa plana by means of acetabuloplasty. Clin Orthop Relat Res 2009;467:608–15.

20. Harris WH. Etiology of osteoarthritis of the hip. Clin Orthop Relat Res 1986;(213):20–33.

21. Ganz R, Gill TJ, Gautier E, et al. Surgical dislocation of the adult hip a technique with full access to the femoral head and acetabulum without the risk of avascular necrosis. J Bone Joint Surg Br 2001;83:1119–24.

22. Ganz R, Parvizi J, Beck M, et al. Femoroacetabular impingement: a cause for osteoarthritis of the hip. Clin Orthop Relat Res 2003;(417):112–20.

23. Anderson LA, Peters CL, Park BB, et al. Acetabular cartilage delamination in femoroacetabular impingement. Risk factors and magnetic resonance imaging diagnosis. J Bone Joint Surg Am 2009;91:305–13.

24. Tannast M, Goricki D, Beck M, et al. Hip damage occurs at the zone of femoroacetabular impingement. Clin Orthop Relat Res 2008;466:273–80.

25. Hastings DE, Parker SM. Protrusio acetabuli in rheumatoid arthritis. Clin Orthop Relat Res 1975;(108):76–83.

26. Wenger DR, Ditkoff TJ, Herring JA, et al. Protrusio acetabuli in Marfan's syndrome. Clin Orthop Relat Res 1980;(147):134–8.

27. Wroblewski BM, Hillman F. Idiopathic protrusio acetabuli. A histological study. Clin Orthop Relat Res 1979;(138):228–30.

28. Clohisy JC, Knaus ER, Hunt DM, et al. Clinical presentation of patients with symptomatic anterior hip impingement. Clin Orthop Relat Res 2009;467:638–44.

29. Mast JW, Brunner RL, Zebrack J. Recognizing acetabular version in the radiographic presentation of hip dysplasia. Clin Orthop Relat Res 2004;(418):48–53.

30. Ezoe M, Naito M, Inoue T. The prevalence of acetabular retroversion among various disorders of the hip. J Bone Joint Surg Am 2006;88:372–9.

31. Li PL, Ganz R. Morphologic features of congenital acetabular dysplasia: one in six is retroverted. Clin Orthop Relat Res 2003;(416):245–53.

32. Tannast M, Zheng G, Anderegg C, et al. Tilt and rotation correction of acetabular version on pelvic radiographs. Clin Orthop Relat Res 2005;438:182–90.

33. Siebenrock KA, Kalbermatten DF, Ganz R. Effect of pelvic tilt on acetabular retroversion: a study of pelves from cadavers. Clin Orthop Relat Res 2003;(407):241–8.

34. Fuchs-Winkelmann S, Peterlein CD, Tibesku CO, et al. Comparison of pelvic radiographs in weight-bearing and supine positions. Clin Orthop Relat Res 2008;466:809–12.

35. Troelsen A, Jacobsen S, Romer L, et al. Weight-bearing anteroposterior pelvic radiographs are recommended in DDH assessment. Clin Orthop Relat Res 2008;466:813–9.

36. Tonnis D. Congenital dysplasia and dislocation of the hip in children and adults. New York: Springer; 1987.

37. Shenton E. Disease in bone and its detection by X-rays. London: Macmillan; 1911.

38. Reynolds D, Lucas J, Klaue K. Retroversion of the acetabulum. A cause of hip pain. J Bone Joint Surg Br 1999;81:281–8.

39. Kakaty DK, Fischer AF, Hosalkar HS, et al. The ischial spine sign: does pelvic tilt and rotation matter? Clin Orthop Relat Res 2010;468:769–74.

40. Kalberer F, Sierra RJ, Madan SS, et al. Ischial spine projection into the pelvis: a new sign for acetabular retroversion. Clin Orthop Relat Res 2008;466:677–83.

41. Beck M, Kalhor M, Leunig M, et al. Hip morphology influences the pattern of damage to the acetabular cartilage: femoroacetabular impingement as a cause of early osteoarthritis of the hip. J Bone Joint Surg Br 2005;87:1012–8.

42. Lequesne MG, Laredo JD. The faux profil (oblique view) of the hip in the standing position. Contribution to the evaluation of osteoarthritis of the adult hip. Ann Rheum Dis 1998;57:676–81.

43. Andren L, von Rosen S. The diagnosis of dislocation of the hip in newborns and the primary results of immediate treatment. Acta Radiol 1958;49:89–95.

44. Murphy S, Deshmukh R. Periacetabular osteotomy: preoperative radiographic predictors of outcome. Clin Orthop Relat Res 2002;(405):168–74.

45. Eijer H, Leunig M, Mahomed MN, et al. Crosstable lateral radiograph for screening of anterior femoral head-neck offset in patients with femoroacetabular impingement. Hip Int 2001;11:37–41.

46. Clohisy JC, Nunley RM, Otto RJ, et al. The frog-leg lateral radiograph accurately visualized hip cam impingement abnormalities. Clin Orthop Relat Res 2007;462:115–21.

47. Notzli HP, Wyss TF, Stoecklin CH, et al. The contour of the femoral head-neck junction as a predictor for the risk of anterior impingement. J Bone Joint Surg Br 2002;84:556–60.

48. Meyer DC, Beck M, Ellis T, et al. Comparison of six radiographic projections to assess femoral head/neck asphericity. Clin Orthop Relat Res 2006;445:181–5.

49. Domayer SE, Ziebarth K, Chan J, et al. Femoroacetabular cam-type impingement: diagnostic sensitivity and specificity of radiographic views compared to radial MRI. Eur J Radiol 2011;80:805–10.

50. Stem ES, O'Connor MI, Kransdorf MJ, et al. Computed tomography analysis of acetabular anteversion and abduction. Skeletal Radiol 2006;35:385–9.

51. Tohtz SW, Sassy D, Matziolis G, et al. CT evaluation of native acetabular orientation and localization: sex-specific data comparison on 336 hip joints. Technol Health Care 2010;18:129–36.

52. Maruyama M, Feinberg JR, Capello WN, et al. The Frank Stinchfield Award: morphologic features of the acetabulum and femur: anteversion angle and implant positioning. Clin Orthop Relat Res 2001;(393):52–65.

53. Anda S, Svenningsen S, Dale LG, et al. The acetabular sector angle of the adult hip determined by computed tomography. Acta Radiol Diagn (Stockh) 1986;27:443–7.

54. Anda S, Terjesen T, Kvistad KA. Computed tomography measurements of the acetabulum in adult dysplastic hips: which level is appropriate? Skeletal Radiol 1991;20:267–71.

55. Fujii M, Nakashima Y, Yamamoto T, et al. Acetabular retroversion in developmental dysplasia of the hip. J Bone Joint Surg Am 2010;92:895–903.

56. Perreira AC, Hunter JC, Laird T, et al. Multilevel measurement of acetabular version using 3-D CT-generated models: implications for hip preservation surgery. Clin Orthop Relat Res 2011;469:552–61.

57. Lubovsky O, Peleg E, Joskowicz L, et al. Acetabular orientation variability and symmetry based on CT scans of adults. Int J Comput Assist Radiol Surg 2010;5:449–54.

58. Klaue K, Wallin A, Ganz R. CT evaluation of coverage and congruency of the hip prior to osteotomy. Clin Orthop Relat Res 1988;(232):15–25.

59. Murphy SB, Kijewski PK, Millis MB, et al. Acetabular dysplasia in the adolescent and young adult. Clin Orthop Relat Res 1990;(261):214–23.

60. Janzen DL, Aippersbach SE, Munk PL, et al. Three-dimensional CT measurement of adult acetabular dysplasia: technique, preliminary results in normal subjects, and potential applications. Skeletal Radiol 1998;27:352–8.

61. Haddad FS, Garbuz DS, Duncan CP, et al. CT evaluation of periacetabular osteotomies. J Bone Joint Surg Br 2000;82:526–31.

62. Ito H, Matsuno T, Hirayama T, et al. Three-dimensional computed tomography analysis of non-osteoarthritic adult acetabular dysplasia. Skeletal Radiol 2009;38:131–9.

63. van Bosse HJ, Lee D, Henderson ER, et al. Pelvic positioning creates error in CT acetabular measurements. Clin Orthop Relat Res 2011;469:1683–91.

64. Dandachli W, Ul Islam S, Tippett R, et al. Analysis of acetabular version in the native hip: comparison between 2D axial CT and 3D CT measurements. Skeletal Radiol 2011;40:877–83.

65. Abel MF, Sutherland DH, Wenger DR, et al. Evaluation of CT scans and 3-D reformatted images for quantitative assessment of the hip. J Pediatr Orthop 1994;14:48–53.

66. Berrington de Gonzalez A, Mahesh M, Kim KP, et al. Projected cancer risks from computed tomographic scans performed in the United States in 2007. Arch Intern Med 2009;169:2071–7.

67. Smith-Bindman R, Lipson J, Marcus R, et al. Radiation dose associated with common computed tomography examinations and the associated

lifetime attributable risk of cancer. Arch Intern Med 2009;169:2078–86.

68. Lang P, Genant HK, Jergesen HE, et al. Imaging of the hip joint. Computed tomography versus magnetic resonance imaging. Clin Orthop Relat Res 1992;(274):135–53.

69. Wenger DE, Kendell KR, Miner MR, et al. Acetabular labral tears rarely occur in the absence of bony abnormalities. Clin Orthop Relat Res 2004; 426:145–50.

70. Plotz GM, Brossmann J, von Knoch M, et al. Magnetic resonance arthrography of the acetabular labrum: value of radial reconstructions. Arch Orthop Trauma Surg 2001;121:450–7.

71. Kubo T, Horii M, Yamaguchi J, et al. Acetabular labrum in hip dysplasia evaluated by radial magnetic resonance imaging. J Rheumatol 2000; 27:1955–60.

72. Dudda M, Albers C, Mamisch TC, et al. Do normal radiographs exclude asphericity of the femoral head-neck junction? Clin Orthop Relat Res 2009; 467:651–9.

73. Rakhra KS, Sheikh AM, Allen D, et al. Comparison of MRI alpha angle measurement planes in femoroacetabular impingement. Clin Orthop Relat Res 2009;467:660–5.

74. Mamisch TC, Bittersohl B, Hughes T, et al. Magnetic resonance imaging of the hip at 3 Tesla: clinical value in femoroacetabular impingement of the hip and current concepts. Semin Musculoskelet Radiol 2008;12:212–22.

75. Czerny C, Hofmann S, Neuhold A, et al. Lesions of the acetabular labrum: accuracy of MR imaging and MR arthrography in detection and staging. Radiology 1996;200:225–30.

76. Leunig M, Werlen S, Ungersbock A, et al. Evaluation of the acetabular labrum by MR arthrography. J Bone Joint Surg Br 1997;79:230–4.

77. Petersilge CA. MR arthrography for evaluation of the acetabular labrum. Skeletal Radiol 2001;30:423–30.

78. Byrd JW, Jones KS. Diagnostic accuracy of clinical assessment, magnetic resonance imaging, magnetic resonance arthrography, and intra-articular injection in hip arthroscopy patients. Am J Sports Med 2004; 32:1668–74.

79. Mintz DN, Hooper T, Connell D, et al. Magnetic resonance imaging of the hip: detection of labral and chondral abnormalities using noncontrast imaging. Arthroscopy 2005;21:385–93.

80. Sundberg TP, Toomayan GA, Major NM. Evaluation of the acetabular labrum at 3.0-T MR imaging compared with 1.5-T MR arthrography: preliminary experience. Radiology 2006;238:706–11.

81. Keeney JA, Peelle MW, Jackson J, et al. Magnetic resonance arthrography versus arthroscopy in the evaluation of articular hip pathology. Clin Orthop Relat Res 2004;(429):163–9.

82. Schmid MR, Notzli HP, Zanetti M, et al. Cartilage lesions in the hip: diagnostic effectiveness of MR arthrography. Radiology 2003;226:382–6.

83. Ulrich-Vinther M, Maloney MD, Schwarz EM, et al. Articular cartilage biology. J Am Acad Orthop Surg 2003;11:421–30.

84. Mosher TJ, Dardzinski BJ. Cartilage MRI T2 relaxation time mapping: overview and applications. Semin Musculoskelet Radiol 2004;8:355–68.

85. Dunn TC, Lu Y, Jin H, et al. T2 relaxation time of cartilage at MR imaging: comparison with severity of knee osteoarthritis. Radiology 2004;232:592–8.

86. David-Vaudey E, Ghosh S, Ries M, et al. T2 relaxation time measurements in osteoarthritis. Magn Reson Imaging 2004;22:673–82.

87. Burstein D, Gray ML. Is MRI fulfilling its promise for molecular imaging of cartilage in arthritis? Osteoarthr Cartil 2006;14:1087–90.

88. Apprich S, Mamisch TC, Welsch GH, et al. Quantitative T2 mapping of the patella at 3.0T is sensitive to early cartilage degeneration, but also to loading of the knee. Eur J Radiol 2012;81(4):e438–43.

89. Nishii T, Shiomi T, Tanaka H, et al. Loaded cartilage T2 mapping in patients with hip dysplasia. Radiology 2010;256:955–65.

90. Bittersohl B, Hosalkar HS, Hughes T, et al. Feasibility of T2* mapping for the evaluation of hip joint cartilage at 1.5T using a three-dimensional (3D), gradient-echo (GRE) sequence: a prospective study. Magn Reson Med 2009;62:896–901.

91. Venn M, Maroudas A. Chemical composition and swelling of normal and osteoarthrotic femoral head cartilage. I. Chemical composition. Ann Rheum Dis 1977;36:121–9.

92. Regatte RR, Akella SV, Borthakur A, et al. Proteoglycan depletion-induced changes in transverse relaxation maps of cartilage: comparison of T2 and T1rho. Acad Radiol 2002;9:1388–94.

93. Regatte RR, Akella SV, Borthakur A, et al. In vivo proton MR three-dimensional T1rho mapping of human articular cartilage: initial experience. Radiology 2003;229:269–74.

94. Gray ML, Burstein D, Kim YJ, et al. 2007 Elizabeth Winston Lanier Award winner. Magnetic resonance imaging of cartilage glycosaminoglycan: basic principles, imaging technique, and clinical applications. J Orthop Res 2008;26:281–91.

95. Burstein D, Velyvis J, Scott KT, et al. Protocol issues for delayed Gd(DTPA)(2-)-enhanced MRI (dGEMRIC) for clinical evaluation of articular cartilage. Magn Reson Med 2001;45:36–41.

96. Tiderius CJ, Jessel R, Kim YJ, et al. Hip dGEMRIC in asymptomatic volunteers and patients with early osteoarthritis: the influence of timing after contrast injection. Magn Reson Med 2007;57:803–5.

97. Kim YJ, Jaramillo D, Millis MB, et al. Assessment of early osteoarthritis in hip dysplasia with delayed

gadolinium-enhanced magnetic resonance imaging of cartilage. J Bone Joint Surg Am 2003;85:1987–92.

98. Cunningham T, Jessel R, Zurakowski D, et al. Delayed gadolinium-enhanced magnetic resonance imaging of cartilage to predict early failure of Bernese periacetabular osteotomy for hip dysplasia. J Bone Joint Surg Am 2006;88:1540–8.

99. Bittersohl B, Steppacher S, Haamberg T, et al. Cartilage damage in femoroacetabular impingement (FAI): preliminary results on comparison of standard diagnostic vs delayed gadolinium-enhanced magnetic resonance imaging of cartilage (dGEMRIC). Osteoarthr Cartil 2009;17:1297–306.

100. Mamisch TC, Kain MS, Bittersohl B, et al. Delayed gadolinium-enhanced magnetic resonance imaging of cartilage (dGEMRIC) in femoacetabular impingement. J Orthop Res 2011;29:1305–11.

101. Zilkens C, Holstein A, Bittersohl B, et al. Delayed gadolinium-enhanced magnetic resonance imaging of cartilage in the long-term follow-up after Perthes disease. J Pediatr Orthop 2010;30:147–53.

102. Zilkens C, Miese F, Bittersohl B, et al. Delayed gadolinium-enhanced magnetic resonance imaging of cartilage (dGEMRIC), after slipped capital femoral epiphysis. Eur J Radiol 2011;79:400–6.

Periacetabular Osteotomy for Hip Preservation

Lisa M. Tibor, MD, Ernest L. Sink, MD*

KEYWORDS

- Hip dysplasia • Hip pain • Periacetabular osteotomy • PAO • Femoroacetabular impingement
- Hip preservation

KEY POINTS

- The Bernese periacetabular osteotomy (PAO) allows for improved position of the weight-bearing acetabular hyaline cartilage. It allows joint medialization and version reorientation while the posterior column is left intact.
- The procedure is indicated in patients who have minimal hip arthrosis and symptomatic hip dysplasia with a concentric hip joint.
- The procedure has a significant learning curve but has a reproducible technique with a low complication rate while prolonging the natural hip joint.
- Acetabular reorientation with a PAO can also improve symptoms from pathologic acetabular retroversion or anteversion.

INTRODUCTION

The goal of any acetabular osteotomy, regardless of the specific technique, is to change the pathologic mechanics of the hip that lead to intra-articular damage, pain, and osteoarthritis.[1] This generally involves improving the coverage of the femoral head and/or changing the orientation of the acetabulum. Reorientation of a dysplastic acetabulum increases the load-bearing surface area of the joint[2] while maintaining or improving joint stability.[3,4] The Bernese PAO was developed by Reinhold Ganz and colleagues in 1983.[5] Compared with other surgical techniques for acetabular reorientation in use at the time, it involves a series of reproducible hexagonal cuts around the acetabulum that leave the posterior column of the pelvis intact. Since the original description, the technique and understanding of the biomechanics have continued to evolve, such that Siebenrock and colleagues wrote in 2001, "Our understanding of what is an optimal correction has improved considerably over time. It is a balancing of the maloriented horseshoe-shaped acetabular cartilage over the femoral head, which leads to an optimal use of a limited area of hyaline cartilage for weight-bearing."[6]

The Bernese PAO has several advantages compared with other acetabular reorientation osteotomies. Specifically, the posterior column of the pelvis remains intact, which maintains the stability of the pelvis and allows early patient mobility. Before the development of the PAO, osteotomy techniques violated the posterior column, requiring either a period of spica cast immobilization or more-extensive pelvic fixation, with an inherent risk of nonunion at the osteotomy site. Because the osteotomy is close to the joint, there is no change in the dimensions of the true pelvis.[7–9] As a result, vaginal childbirth is still safe for these patients, which is not the case for adult patients who have had double or triple pelvic osteotomies. The proximity of the osteotomy to the joint also allows for potentially powerful correction of the bony mechanics.[10,11] In particular, because the joint is medialized, the lever arm of the abductors improves and the joint reactive forces decrease. Finally, because all of the osteotomy cuts are made from the inner aspect of the pelvis, the

Center for Hip Pain and Preservation, Hospital for Special Surgery, 535 East 70th Street, New York, NY 10021, USA
* Corresponding author.
E-mail address: sinke@hss.edu

Orthop Clin N Am 43 (2012) 343–357
doi:10.1016/j.ocl.2012.05.011
0030-5898/12/$ – see front matter © 2012 Elsevier Inc. All rights reserved.

orthopedic.theclinics.com

abductors can be preserved. The curved or spherical PAO, which is more common in Asia, has some of the same advantages. With this technique, however, the osteotomy fragment is smaller; it may be more susceptible to osteonecrosis and the medialization of the hip center may be more limited.[5,12] Nonetheless, the Bernese PAO is technically complex and there is a substantial surgical learning curve to the procedure.[11,13,14]

ANATOMY

The original technique was developed in 1983 and published in 1988 with 1-year follow-up results from the first 75 patients.[5] The bone cuts were developed based on knowledge of the blood supply to the acetabular fragment (**Figs. 1** and **2**). Briefly, the pelvis is approached through either a direct anterior or modified Smith-Petersen approach, taking care to preserve the abductors. The ischium is cut just inferior to the infracotyloid notch; the pubis is cut adjacent to the acetabulum; and the supra-acetabular osteotomy begins in the

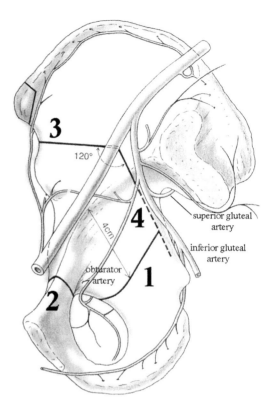

Fig. 2. Drawing of the acetabular blood supply to the internal pelvic surface and sequence of osteotomies: (1) ischial osteotomy, (2) pubic osteotomy, (3) supra-acetabular osteotomy, and (4) retroacetabular osteotomy. (*Reprinted from* Leunig M, Siebenrock KA, Ganz R. Instructional Course Lecture, American Academy of Orthopedic Surgeons. Rationale of periacetabular osteotomy and background work. J Bone Joint Surg Am 2001;83:437–47; with permission.)

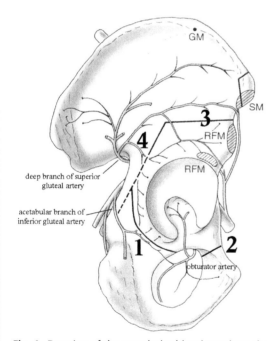

Fig. 1. Drawing of the acetabular blood supply to the external pelvic surface and the sequence of osteotomies: (1) ischial osteotomy, (2) pubic osteotomy, (3) supra-acetabular osteotomy, and (4) retroacetabular osteotomy. GM, gluteus medius tubercle; RFM, rectus femoris muscle (direct and indirect) heads; SM, sartorius muscle attachment. (*Reprinted from* Leunig M, Siebenrock KA, Ganz R. Instructional course lecture, American Academy of Orthopedic Surgeons. Rationale of periacetabular osteotomy and background work. J Bone Joint Surg Am 2001;83:437–47; with permission.)

region of the anterior superior iliac spine (ASIS). Just lateral to the acetabular brim, the cut is angled 120° to meet the ischial osteotomy. The endosteal blood supply to the fragment is disrupted by the osteotomy, but fragment perfusion is maintained by 2 branches of the superior gluteal artery, the acetabular branch of the inferior gluteal artery and the acetabular branch of the obturator artery.[15] There is additional contribution of the capsular blood supply, unless the osteotomy is performed too close to the capsule.[16]

Investigation of the effects of PAO in various patient populations has been reported in the literature. Many patients with dysplasia are young, female, and of childbearing age. The impact of the PAO on the dimensions of the true pelvis, pregnancy, and childbirth has been studied.[7–9] Study results reveal no change in the anteroposterior (AP) inlet, midpelvis, bispinous diameter, or transverse inlet measurements after PAO.[7–9] Clinically, women who have had prior PAOs report vaginal deliveries and cesarean sections for reasons unrelated to the osteotomy.[8,17] In one series, the rates of cesarean section were increased above population averages.[8] Although firm conclusions could not be drawn, the increase was attributed in part to obstetrician concerns for the patients' prior osteotomies. Patients who had been sexually active after a PAO reported both increased and decreased sexual activity secondary to changes in pain and range of motion after the surgery.[17] Patients who became pregnant after having a PAO reported back and hip pain during pregnancy that resolved after childbirth.[17] The authors of this study of PAO patients reporting pain with pregnancy observed a correlation of patient pain and range of motion to acetabular retroversion and probable impingement.[17]

EVOLUTION OF THE TECHNIQUE

Since its initial description, the surgical technique has undergone various modifications. Although a Smith-Petersen approach to the anterior aspect of the pelvis was part of the original technique,[5] the abductors were stripped from the iliac wing to perform the supra-acetabular osteotomy. This has evolved such that the abductors are largely left intact when the osteotomy is performed.[1,13,18] In addition to preserving the abductor function, protecting the abductors preserves the obturator, superior and inferior gluteal arteries, and the capsular contribution to acetabular perfusion, decreasing the risk of acetabular osteonecrosis.[15,16] Initially, the bone cuts were performed from both sides of the iliac wing; however, to preserve the abductors, the bone cuts have been changed and are now mostly performed from the inner aspect of the pelvis.[5,13,15] More recently, it has become apparent that hip flexion strength is decreased for up to 2 years postoperatively.[19] Thus, a rectus-sparing approach, which leaves the direct and indirect heads of the rectus femoris attached to the ilium, has been advocated for preserving hip flexor strength.

The recognition that femoroacetabular impingement (FAI) could be responsible for continued pain after a PAO was an important development.[20] The femoral head in a dysplastic hip is known to have an elliptical shape with decreased head-neck offset[21] and lateral flattening from a hypertrophic gluteus minimus.[22] When the acetabulum is reoriented such that there is excess lateral or anterior coverage, FAI can occur. As a result, an arthrotomy has been incorporated into the surgical technique for evaluation of impingement. When necessary, a femoral-head neck osteoplasty is performed through the arthrotomy.[20] Better recognition of acetabular version during the correction also helps minimize FAI because the acetabulum can be excessively retroverted, resulting

in pincer-type FAI[13,17,23] or undercoverage of the posterior aspect of the hip.[2,13]

Other modifications to the original surgical technique have been described and adopted to varying degrees. One modification was the description of a 2-incision technique so that the ischial osteotomy could be performed under direct visualization.[24,25] The disadvantage of this technique, as it was described, is that it requires takedown of the external rotators posteriorly.[25] This may endanger the medial femoral circumflex artery, which is the primary blood supply to the femoral head.[26] There may also be difficulty with the correction and assessing fragment version because of patient positioning and loss of some of the soft tissue tension.[25] Additional variations to the technique include intraoperative fluoroscopy to judge the position of the osteotomies[27] and minimally invasive incisions.[28,29]

Recently, some investigators have also begun performing arthroscopy at the time of PAO to evaluate the articular cartilage and refix or stabilize the labrum.[30] The clinical outcome of labral refixation in this setting is, as yet, unknown.[30]

BIOMECHANICS

Computer modeling and finite element analysis haves allowed the biomechanical effects of PAO to be quantified. On average, a PAO increases the load-bearing surface of the joint by approximately 50%, with a range of 35% to 70% depending on the degree of correction. This is comparable to the load-bearing surface for normal control patients.[2] The increased femoral head coverage causes improved load distribution, with near-normal contact stresses observed in 3-D finite element analysis.[31] Contact pressure analysis has also revealed that the amount of correction required for an optimal decrease in load varies among patients.[32] For patients with a typical pattern of dysplasia requiring lateral and anterior coverage, the largest reduction in cartilage contact pressures occurred when the fragment was adducted and extended.[32]

Acetabular reorientation also improves hip stability. The dysplastic hip is both statically and dynamically unstable, with superior, posterior, and lateral movement of the femoral head with walking, compared with hips with normal morphology.[3] In a recent study, the dynamic instability was restored to near-normal values after acetabular reorientation.[3] In a computational model of hip dysplasia, lateral hip stability improved to normal values when the center-edge angle measured 25° to 30°. The same model observed that anterior and posterior femoral head stability correlated with the degree of acetabular version.[4]

Improvement in hip biomechanics can also be observed clinically. For example, redistribution of the acetabular load may result in a change in the bone density. As such, acetabular bone density after PAO has been assessed with both CT and dual energy x-ray absorptiometry (DEXA) scanning. Anteromedial bone density was found increased 2 years postoperatively,[33] but there was no change in lateral bone density. An underpowered study using DEXA scanning to assess acetabular bone density 2.5 years after PAO failed to observe a difference in density. The investigators concluded that DEXA scanning did not provide enough resolution to adequately assess bony changes after a PAO.[34] Nonetheless, the redistribution of load has some effect on the subchondral bone, as evidenced by acetabular cysts that healed after acetabular reorientation.[35] Furthermore, the degree of healing also correlated with the degree of correction and the clinical outcome score.[35] Close examination of the articular surface revealed that cartilage thickness and the shape of the articular surface are both preserved in short-term follow-up (1–2.5 years).[36,37] Finally, gait and strength comparative analysis preoperatively and postoperatively reveals that abductor strength was better 1 year postoperatively but flexion was still weak compared with healthy controls.[19] This may be the reason that the increased knee flexion seen in preoperative gait analysis improved but did not entirely resolve.[38]

INDICATIONS AND CONTRAINDICATIONS

The most accepted indication for acetabular reorientation is mild to moderate symptomatic dysplasia.[1,5,6,11,14,18,30,39–41] Initially, there was controversy about the degree of dysplasia and concomitant femoral head deformity that can be adequately addressed with a PAO[12]; it was believed that severely subluxed hips would require salvage osteotomies instead.[12] Subsequently, good outcomes have been published for more severe deformities and the indications have been expanded. Thus, dysplasia secondary to Legg-Calvé-Perthes disease and dysplasia secondary to flaccid and spastic neuromuscular disorders are considered appropriate indications for PAO.[42–45] Global acetabular retroversion causing impingement is also considered an indication for PAO, particularly if the retroversion is associated with posterior wall deficiency or posterior instability.[46,47]

There may also be a role for acetabular reorientation in patients with borderline dysplasia (center-edge angle of Wiberg of 20°–25°) and clinically symptomatic instability. This occurs most often in the setting of increased femoral and/or acetabular anteversion (Fig. 3) and primarily manifests as iliopsoas or abductor fatigue symptoms.[48,49] Although there are biomechanical data demonstrating that hip stability and acetabular load are related to acetabular version,[4] there are as yet no clinical outcomes data for this patient population.

Midterm and long-term follow-up have established that the most predictable outcomes are in patients under 35 years old at the time of surgery[50–52] with little to no arthritis (Tönnis grade 0 or 1) on plain radiographs.[51,53] Good results have, however, been reported for patients over age 35 or 40, even in early series,[5,52] with the caveat that the hip was well preserved and concentric on preoperative imaging.

Study results of PAO in patients with preoperative arthrosis reveal that Tönnis grades 2 and 3 are greater predictors of failure.[51,53–55] A cost-efficacy analysis found that total hip arthroplasty was preferable for Tönnis grade 3 arthrosis but that in grade 1 or 2 arthrosis, PAO was the more appropriate treatment.[56] Although the presence of grade 2 or 3 arthrosis is a predictor of failure, some patients with this degree of arthrosis show improved outcomes scores and relatively preserved joint space in midterm follow-up.[54] Thus, although arthrosis is a relative contraindication to PAO, PAO may be preferable to total hip arthroplasty in certain younger patients.

Contraindications to PAO include incongruence on functional radiographs (abduction and internal rotation images or flexion false profile images), which indicates potentially worse congruency after acetabular reorientation and is thus a predictor of worse outcomes.[51] This can occur in nonspherical femoral heads or when the acetabular radius is smaller than the femoral head radius.[1] PAO is also contraindicated in young patients (<10 or 11 years of age) because of the risk of injury to the triradiate cartilage, through which the PAO bone cuts are made. In series of patients with post-traumatic acetabular dysplasia secondary to an acetabular fracture and subsequent growth disturbance, the oldest affected patients were approximately 10 years of age at the time of the fracture.[57,58] Significant growth disturbances have not been observed in adolescents with open triradiate cartilage who sustain acetabular fractures.[57,58] Thus, there seems little risk of injury to the triradiate cartilage after age 10 or 11, which is the lower age limit for a PAO.

PREOPERATIVE PLANNING

The history and physical examination should focus on determining whether a patient's symptoms are primarily from dysplasia and static overload, from FAI, or from both. Pain originating from the spine, pelvis, or muscle should be ruled out as part of

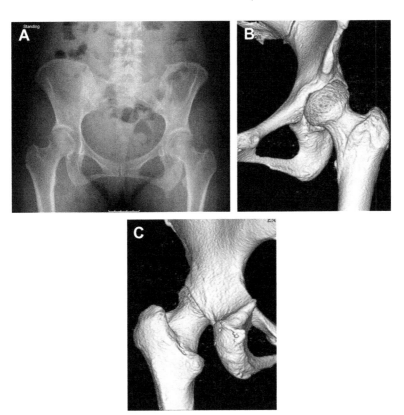

Fig. 3. (*A*) AP hip radiograph of the hips indicating extreme anteversion with a posterior wall lateral to the center of the femoral head and deficient anterior wall coverage. (*B*) A CT scan indicating no acetabular coverage of the anterior femoral head. (*C*) A CT scan indicating excessive posterior joint coverage.

the initial evaluation. Symptoms characteristic of dysplasia include pain independent of motion and peritrochanteric muscular fatigue after standing or prolonged periods of walking.[1] Symptoms more characteristic of FAI include sharp anteromedial groin pain and pain with prolonged sitting.[5] Patients with dysplasia and an acetabular rim lesion, however, may present with sharp anterior groin pain. On examination, patients with dysplasia and true abductor weakness may have a Trendelenburg gait and Trendelenburg sign. Full or increased hip range of motion should be expected for patients with normal acetabular cartilage. Also, when deciding between FAI and dysplasia of the hip, patients with instability have more hip flexion and internal rotation at 90° of flexion. They may also have a positive apprehension test (pain with extension and external rotation). Because the acetabulum is often anteriorly deficient, these patients may also have psoas irritation or snapping.[1]

Initial radiographs should include a standing AP pelvis radiograph, 45° or 90° Dunn lateral view, a false profile view, and a functional view with the affected hip abducted and internally rotated. The AP pelvis radiograph is used to assess lateral coverage and acetabular version; it is important that the radiograph be obtained with the pelvis in neutral flexion and rotation.[59] In the neutral position, the obturator foramen and teardrops appear symmetric and the coccyx is directly in line with the pubic symphysis.[59] The distance between the coccyx and pubic symphysis is a marker of pelvic tilt and measures 1 cm to 3 cm in a correctly obtained radiograph.[59] The Dunn lateral is used to assess the femoral head-neck offset. In patients with insufficient offset, there may be coexistent FAI and dysplasia; furthermore, these patients may have symptoms of FAI after acetabular reorientation. The false profile view is used to evaluate anterior acetabular coverage, whereas the abduction and internal rotation view is used to assess hip congruency after a potential correction.

CT scanning serves as a useful addition to plain radiographs for preoperative planning.[13] 3-D reconstructions improve the assessment of acetabular version and socket depth. In addition, the prominence of the anterior inferior iliac spine (AIIS) can be assessed with a CT scan (**Fig. 4**). After reorientation of the acetabulum, a prominent AIIS can contribute to extra-articular impingement. An MRI

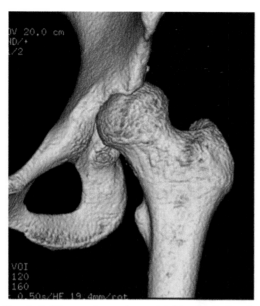

Fig. 4. A CT scan of a patient with hip dysplasia. The prominence of the AIIS is obvious on this image. After reorientation of the acetabulum, this prominent AIIS can cause extra-articular impingement.

provides a better evaluation of the labrum and cartilage. For patients with mild or questionable pre-existing arthrosis, cartilage-specific sequences, such as delayed gadolinium-enhanced MRI of cartilage (dGEMRIC), T1rho, or T2 mapping, as described in a previous article,[60] may play a role in surgical decision-making. Pre-existing intra-articular damage is a negative prognostic factor, which may have an impact on surgical decision-making and is important to take into account in managing patient expectations.

AUTHORS' PREFERRED TECHNIQUE

PAO can be performed with either general anesthesia or under combined spinal-epidural anesthesia and sedation. One advantage of the spinal-epidural anesthesia is that the epidural can be left in place for postoperative pain relief. Patients may opt to predonate 1 unit of autologous blood and receive it back the morning after surgery. Intraoperatively, a cell saver is also used.

If adjuvant arthroscopy is performed for labral repair or débridement and cartilage assessment, the arthroscopy is performed first with the patient on a traction table using a standard technique. The combination of arthroscopy and PAO in the same setting has been previously described,[30] but outcomes data are not yet available. Nonetheless, PAO patients with intact labra had better long-term outcomes scores and a lower risk of arthrosis progression.[41,47]

For the PAO, patients are positioned supine on a standard radiolucent table. All bony prominences are well padded and the ipsilateral arm is positioned such that it does not impede the placement of the chisel or screws intraoperatively. The senior author's preference is to place it in a 90°–90° position of abduction and external rotation. The entire operative leg is prepped and draped. The incision is slightly curved lateral to the ASIS and the tensor-sartorius interval (**Fig. 5**). The fascia over the tensor fascia lata is opened to expose the medial aspect of the muscle to its insertion at the pelvis between the ASIS and the AIIS. The deep lateral rectus fascia is opened and the rectus is retracted medially. The lateral floor of the rectus fascia is then visualized. Often the transverse vessels of the lateral femoral artery are visualized deep to this fascia, which marks the distal extent of the exposure. Opening the floor of the rectus fascia then exposes the lateral aspect of the iliocapsularis muscle. The interval between the hip capsule and the iliocapsularis is developed as the iliocapsularis is retracted medially. Next the ASIS is osteotomized and reflected medially, preserving the sartorius attachment on the osteotomized fragment. Care is taken near the ASIS because proximally the lateral femoral cutaneous nerve

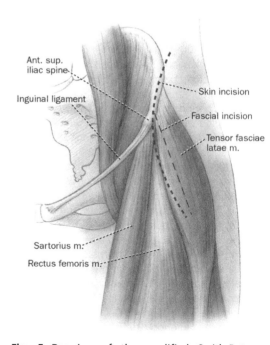

Fig. 5. Drawing of the modified Smith-Petersen approach for PAO. (*Reprinted from* Clohisy JC, Barrett SE, Gordon JE, et al. Periacetabular osteotomy in the treatment of severe acetabular dysplasia. Surgical technique. J Bone Joint Surg Am 2006;88(Suppl 1): 65–83; with permission.)

emerges within 5 cm of and medial to the ASIS[61] and can be injured during the approach.[13] Proximally, the external oblique aponeurosis is sharply incised and the iliacus is elevated subperiosteally and medially off the iliac wing. At this point in the procedure, flexing the leg to 45° decreases the soft tissue tension and facilitates further dissection.

Because of reports of prolonged hip flexor weakness after PAO,[19] the direct and indirect head of the rectus can be left attached (rectus-sparing modification) and retracted laterally during the capsular exposure. At this point, the iliocapsularis can be visualized. The iliocapsularis muscle, which is directly attached to the anterior capsule, is generally hypertrophied because of its role as a secondary stabilizer in the dysplastic hip.[62] It should be carefully elevated off the capsule and reflected medially. This brings the anterior aspect of the joint into view. A pointed Hohman retractor can be placed on the superior pubic ramus to facilitate this.

Next, the iliopsoas bursa is identified by gentle elevation and medial retraction of the iliacus, iliocapsularis, and rectus (if the rectus was taken off its insertion). Once this bursa is opened, a retractor is placed deep to the iliopsoas tendon to allow gentle medial retraction of the tendon. Once the lateral aspect of the superior pubic ramus is visualized, the subperiosteal dissection of the ilium can be extended to the quadrilateral plate. This allows a blunt Hohman to be placed on the ischial

spine and enables visualization of the inner table of the pelvis. The sciatic nerve emerges from the greater sciatic notch, which is close to the intrapelvic retractor. Electromyographic studies indicate that nerve irritation does occur intraoperatively; thus, it is critical that care be taken with retractor placement.[63]

The interval between the iliopsoas tendon and the joint capsule is developed medially, allowing access to the ischium for the first osteotomy. Large curved scissors are used to determine the width of the ischium. A Judet or false profile view of the acetabulum is obtained with intraoperative fluoroscopy. A specially curved or angled chisel is then passed into the interval and used to make the first cut. The osteotomy can be performed using fluoroscopic visualization and begins just inferior to the infracotyloid notch, extending posteriorly for 15 mm to 20 mm toward the base of the ischial spine (**Fig. 6**). The resistance between the femoral head and the chisel provides proprioceptive feedback about the osteotome position. When the femoral head is subluxed, this resistance is lost and additional care must be taken to ensure that the osteotome and osteotomy remain outside of the joint. Intra-articular propagation of the ischial osteotomy is a significant problem. Care should be taken to avoid this because of the potential for joint surface incongruity and because of the potential for damage to the acetabular branch of the obturator

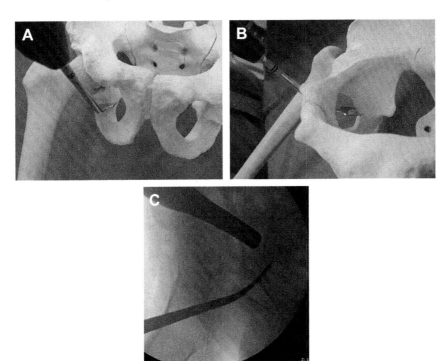

Fig. 6. (*A, B*) Location of the insertion point of the chisel for the ischial cut below the acetabulum as shown on a pelvic model. (*C*) Intraoperative fluoroscopic false profile view showing the location of the ischial cut.

artery, which is one of the sources of perfusion for the fragment.[13,15] The lateral portion of the ischial osteotomy is close to the sciatic nerve; the nerve is at risk if the osteotome slips laterally. The nerve can be protected to a certain extent by placing the leg in abduction and extension and directing the osteotome medially.

Attention is then directed to the pubic osteotomy. The superior pubic ramus is dissected subperiosteally and a pointed Hohman retractor is hammered into the ramus medial to the osteotomy for visualization. Blunt retractors are placed around the bone to protect the obturator nerve, which runs on the inferior aspect of the ramus.[64] The cut is made just medial to the pectineal eminence and perpendicular to the bone, which is generally approximately 45° to the plane of the table (**Fig. 7**).

Attention is turned to the supra-acetabular osteotomy. The abductors are tunneled only at the level of the osteotomy, and a blunt Hohman retractor is placed in the greater sciatic notch. Additional soft tissue is elevated off the quadrilateral surface. There are 2 portions to the supra-acetabular cuts; the first passes through the iliac wing and the second is retroacetabular, meeting up with the ischial osteotomy. Both are often performed under direct and fluoroscopic visualization and can be made with either an oscillating saw or osteotome. Before beginning the cuts, a target mark or hole is made approximately 1 cm lateral to the pelvic brim often in line with the apex of the sciatic notch on false profile views. At this mark the angle of the osteotomy changes. The retroacetabular cut angles 120° from the supra-acetabular cut and is directed toward the first ischial cut (**Fig. 8**). The anatomy of the quadrilateral surface and the potential for one of

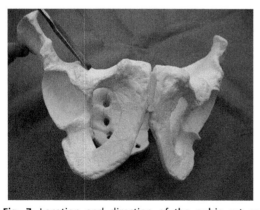

Fig. 7. Location and direction of the pubic cut as shown on a model pelvis. The angle of approximately 45° at the medial border of the pubic eminence will allow the cut to exit just medial to the hip joint in the obturator foramen. The obturator nerve and vessels will need to be protected.

the osteotomies to extend intra-articularly has been analyzed.[65] To obtain an appropriate distance between the supra-acetabular cut and the quadrilateral surface, the initial cut begins in the region of the ASIS osteotomy, approximately 1 cm anterior to the greater sciatic notch.[65] In cases of severe dysplasia, there is an increased risk of the supra-acetabular cut extending into the joint. The consequences can be catastrophic because incongruity in the weightbearing dome of the acetabulum leads to rapid osteoarthrosis.[13]

Depending on a patient's anatomy, the retroacetabular osteotomy is performed with either a straight or curved osteotome. This extends along the posterior column to meet the ischial osteotomy. The cut should be just posterior to the midpoint of the width of the posterior column, defined as the area between the hip joint and the sciatic notch. The osteotome is angled slightly from anterior to posterior to avoid the posterior part of the joint. A useful fluoroscopic technique is to see a perfect lateral image of the osteotome on false profile view when beginning the osteotomy (see **Fig. 8**). Once the osteotomy is completed medially, the lateral cortex is osteotomized as a controlled fracture. This is undertaken to protect the sciatic nerve, which is directly inferior to the lateral cortex and would be at risk if the osteotomes were used to complete the lateral osteotomy. Fluoroscopy is used to ensure that the retroacetabular osteotomy meets the ischial osteotomy. Once the medial aspects of the osteotomy are performed, the posterolarereral cortex where the iliac and the posterior column osteotomies meet can be cut with an angled osteotome, which also allows more fragment mobilization. At this point there is some risk of the osteotomy propagating into the sciatic notch, with subsequent discontinuity of the posterior column.[13] Although this may ultimately be of little consequence, it does compromise the stability of the healing fragment and the patient must remain non–weight bearing until evidence of fragment healing is seen.

When all of the cuts have been made, a Schanz pin is placed in the acetabular fragment at the AIIS, angled posterior between the inner and outer tables of the pelvis. This facilitates fragment mobilization and control of the fragment during correction. At this time, the fragment should move freely. This is important, because if it does not, the soft tissue or bony hinging hinders the correction and limits medialization of the joint. For classic dysplasia, lateral and anterior correction is essential; thus, the fragment should be adducted and flexed. Nonetheless, the correction should be individualized for each patient and based on the anatomy and information from the preoperative radiographs. Once a preliminary correction has

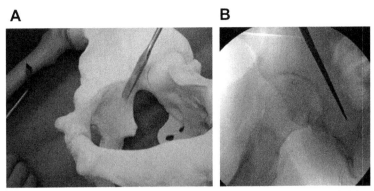

Fig. 8. (*A*) Location and direction of the posterior column cut shown on a pelvic model. (*B*) Intraoperative fluoroscopic false profile view highlighting the posterior column cut. The chisel is oriented at a right angle to the x-ray beam and directed toward the ischial cut. Note that the location of the cut sufficiently posterior to the hip joint and anterior to the sciatic notch.

been obtained, the fragment is fixed with 2-mm Kirschner wires and evaluated fluoroscopically. There are 5 parameters to assess intraoperatively[66]:

1. The sourcil: this should be horizontal but not negative,[13] with the goal of balancing the sourcil over the femoral head.
2. Center edge angle and lateral coverage: the center edge angle should be between 25-35°, with at least 80% lateral coverage of the femoral head.
3. Medial translation of the hip center: the hip center should be slightly medialized to improve joint reactive forces. Excessive medialization, however, can lead to iatrogenic protrusio.[13]
4. Position of the teardrop and ilioischial line: the teardrop should be more medial than previously, reflecting medialization of the joint.
5. Acetabular version: the anterior and posterior walls should meet at the lateral edge of the joint. A crossover sign indicates that the fragment has been flexed too far forward, which results in acetabular retroversion and can contribute to postoperative FAI.

Once a satisfactory correction has been obtained, 3.5-mm or 4.5-mm cortical screws can be placed for definitive fixation. The senior author prefers 4 supra-acetabular screws placed from posterior to anterior in the iliac crest (**Fig. 9**) because this facilitates subsequent hardware removal. In certain cases, a front-to-back transverse screw, can add extra stabilization. The original fixation described by Ganz and colleagues[5] and still used commonly consists of 2 posterior to anterior screws and one posteriorly directed transverse screw placed at the AIIS. Biomechanical analysis of different 3-screw constructs found that constructs with the transverse screw were stiffer[67] and seem to have higher loads to failure.[67,68] The biomechanical effect of a fourth screw is not known. If there are any concerns about fragment stability, integrity of the posterior column, or bone quality, it is reasonable to reinforce the fixation with pelvic reconstruction plates.

Once the correction is obtained and stable, any potential impingement is addressed. Hip range of motion in flexion and internal and external rotation is evaluated. An anterior capsulotomy to evaluate

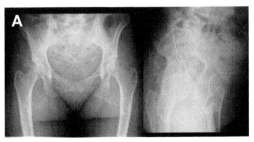
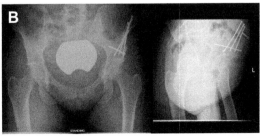

Fig. 9. (*A*) Preoperative AP radiographs of a patient with symptomatic hip dysplasia. (*B*) Postoperative AP and false profile radiograph after a PAO. The goals of balancing the sourcil over the femoral head, improving the lateral and anterior CE angle, medialization of the joint center, and appropriate version of the acetabulum have been achieved.

for impingement is routinely performed to evaluate any potential impingement. Depending on the proximal femoral anatomy, a femoral neck osteoplasty can be performed, particularly if there are any limits to motion. In addition, any restrictions in motion or impingement from the AIIS can be assed and bone from the AIIS can be resected if it is causing impingement. The capsule is then repaired with absorbable suture. The ASIS osteotomy is refixed with a 3.5-mm cortical screw and the remainder of the wound is closed in a layered fashion.

Postoperatively, patients remain in the hospital for 3 to 6 days for pain control and mobilization. Patients are allowed to be toe-touch weight-bearing with crutches for the first 4 to 6 weeks. Weight bearing is limited because load-to-failure testing of the screw constructs found that ultimate failure can occur with loads as low as 1.27-times body weight.[67] In addition, loss of correction has occurred in patients who began weight bearing too soon after surgery.[6,13] Gentle continuous passive motion is used in the hospital to limit adhesion formation and to reassure patients that the hip can move normally. To reduce the risk of thrombosis, mechanical sequential compression devices are used. Depending on patient risk factors, aspirin or other chemoprophylaxis may also be considered. The overall incidence of venous thrombosis after PAO is low (0.94%).[69] In otherwise low-risk patients, the complications of Lovenox or other chemoprophylaxis includes prolonged wound drainage, hematoma, and bleeding, which largely outweigh the risk of deep vein thrombosis or pulmonary embolus.[69]

RESULTS

Early, midterm, and long-term outcomes of PAO have been reported.[5,6,11,12,19,28,29,41–47,50–53] Most patients have significantly improved outcomes scores.[11] Nonetheless, 10% to 12% of patients have fair outcomes that are not related to known predictors of failure.[51]

The presence of arthrosis is the most well-known predictor of failure. For patients with mild to moderate arthrosis (grade 0–1), Harris hip scores improve in early follow-up.[11,53] Long-term follow-up reveals 75% survivorship in this group at 20 years, often with at least one grade of radiographic progression of arthrosis,[50] a mild limp, and decreased range of motion. In a series of patients with a PAO on one side and more advanced arthrosis requiring total hip arthroplasty on the contralateral side, the patients noted increased recovery and difficulty after the PAO but generally preferred the side with the PAO.[70] In contrast, PAO patients with moderate to severe arthrosis (grade 2–3) are at an increased risk of early failure and conversion to total hip

arthroplasty.[53,55] Compared with other patient subgroups undergoing PAO, some patients with moderate to severe arthrosis had worse outcome scores 2 years postoperatively.[53] The long-term survivorship of PAO in this group is 13% at 20 years. Given these results, moderate to severe arthrosis is considered a contraindication to PAO, particularly because it can also increase the difficulty of subsequent arthroplasty.[71]

Survival until total hip arthroplasty varies with the patient population and ranges from 4 months to 14 years. A systematic review of PAO outcomes found that conversion rates ranged from 0% to 14% of patients.[11] Survivorship rates generally declined with time, with 90% survivorship at 5 years, 82% survivorship at 9 years, and 60% survivorship at 20 years.[50,72] The caveat to these results is that these represent some of the first patients who underwent PAO, 24% of whom had arthrosis preoperatively. In general, however, these results are better than those seen for untreated dysplasia.[73]

Outcomes have been reported for several other patient subgroups. Patients who underwent prior acetabular or femoral osteotomies had good radiographic correction of the acetabulum. Nonetheless, the surgeries were more complex, with higher complication rates, less improvement in Harris hip scores, and potentially higher failure rates in short-term to midterm follow-up.[64,74] Similarly, good outcomes have been reported for patients with severe acetabular and femoral deformities, although the cases are more technically complex and have a higher risk of complications.[12,42]

Adolescents undergoing PAO demonstrated similar improvement in outcomes scores compared with adult series.[19] For older patients, however, outcomes are less predictable. In a recent series, age was an increased risk factor for failure.[51] Patients older than 40 at the time of PAO had a 24% arthroplasty conversion rate 5 years postoperatively,[52] with 50% of Tönnis grade 2 hips requiring conversion due to increased postoperative pain.[52] The majority of patients (76%), however, had not required arthroplasty 5 years postoperatively and had improved Harris hip scores and WOMAC pain scores.[52] In series of 40-year-old and 50 year-old Japanese patients undergoing acetabular reorientation via spherical osteotomy, the improvement in outcomes scores is similar to that for younger patients.[75,76] These patients, however, were carefully selected, with minimal to no arthrosis and having close-to-ideal body weight.

HIP ARTHROSCOPY AND PAO

In general, hip arthroscopy should only be used as an adjuvant therapy with PAO for patients with symptomatic hip dysplasia. There is one study that showed short-term improvement in patients with hip dysplasia who underwent arthroscopic repair of labral tears[77]; however, this should be interpreted with caution. Hip arthroscopy without bony correction of dysplasia may not resolve symptoms and may potentially result in femoral head subluxation, continued symptoms, or more rapid progression of osteoarthritis.[71,78] Furthermore, for portal access and intra-articular arthroscopic procedures, the hip capsule must be incised, which may severely destabilize the dysplastic hip.[78] In instances where patients with dysplasia choose to undergo arthroscopy instead of PAO, they should be counseled accordingly about the potential risks (discussed previously) and followed regularly for continued symptoms, instability, or progression of arthrosis.

Many surgeons use hip arthroscopy as an adjuvant treatment with PAO to manage intra-articular pathology and mechanical symptoms due to labral tears or chondral flaps. It has been shown that labral tears are present in 65% to 77% of patients who have hip dysplasia.[30,79] There are not enough long-term outcomes to clarify whether labral repair or débridement in conjunction with a PAO improves overall outcomes compared with osteotomy alone. Nonetheless, given what is known about the biomechanical function of the labrum,[80–87] for patients with clearly detached labral tears on preoperative MRI, it is the authors' preference to carry out arthroscopic labral repair at the same time as PAO (**Fig. 10**).

PAO FOR MILD DYSPLASIA AND FAI

As understanding of the pathomechanics of hip pain advances and the etiology of structural injury to the hip is elucidated, the indications for redirectional acetabular osteotomy may potentially be expanded. Traditionally, the indications for PAO have been largely radiographic and based on the AP pelvis radiograph. Specifically, the most widely accepted role PAO was for patients with a lateral center-edge angle measuring less than 20° and lateral subluxation, as evidenced by a break in Shenton line. As diagnostic imaging and understanding of complex hip disorders evolve, it is likely that the pathology and symptoms resulting from subtle instability will be recognized more often. As a result, the indications for a redirectional osteotomy may be expanded. One example of this is an anteverting osteotomy for FAI occurring in the setting of global acetabular retroversion.[46] There are also patients who have symptoms and labral injury from excessive acetabular anteversion. These symptoms can be alleviated by reorienting

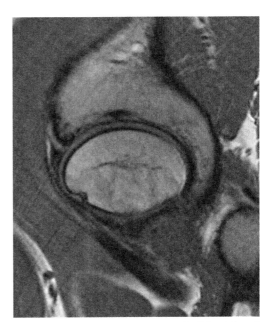

Fig. 10. A sagittal MRI cut showing the labral detachment from the anterior-superior acetabular bone. The labrum is otherwise intact; therefore, arthroscopic labral fixation to the acetabular rim was performed concurrently with the PAO.

the acetabulum to obtain more anterior coverage of the hip (see **Fig. 3**). Similarly, patients with severe femoral anteversion may be symptomatic because of the relative anterior undercoverage, resulting in increased stress on the anterior acetabular rim and labrum. These patients may also benefit from a PAO to increase the anterior acetabular coverage (**Fig. 11**. Reinforcing these ideas are biomechanical data demonstrating that hip stability and acetabular load are related to acetabular version.[4] These ideas are new, however, and there are no clinical outcomes data yet for this patient population.

COMPLICATIONS

The risks and type of complications are generally related to surgical learning curve.[11,13,14] Overall, the complication rate after PAO ranges from 11% to 45%, depending on the series and the learning curve.[51]

Injury to the lateral femoral cutaneous nerve is common, with severity of the injury ranging from transient paresthesias to innocuous numbness to painful neuralgia or neuromas.[13] The incidence of other neurologic complications is much less. Intraoperative electromyography indicates that nerve irritation occurs during surgery, and, accordingly, transient peroneal nerve palsies are not unusual.[51] Injury to the sciatic nerve, secondary to posterior

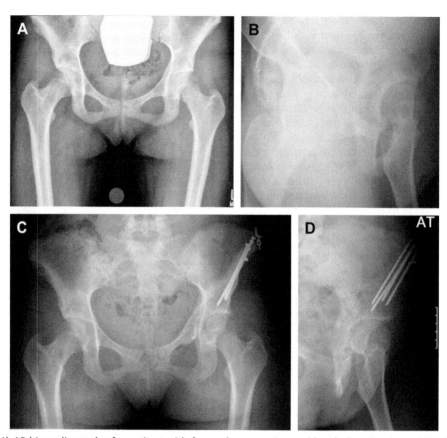

Fig. 11. (*A*) AP hip radiograph of a patient with femoral anteversion and borderline dysplasia. (*B*) False profile indicating poor anterior coverage. (*C*) AP and (*D*) false profile after PAO.

bone fragments, has also been reported.[13] Vascular complications are less common. Before the widespread adoption of the modified Smith-Petersen approach, arterial thrombosis was reported with the ilioinguinal approach.[13,28] There is a report of a patient who had previous pelvic surgery requiring embolization for uncontrolled bleeding from an unnamed vessel, thought to be neovascularization from the prior surgery.[64]

Osteonecrosis of the acetabular fragment is rare but has been reported in a patient with severe dysplasia and a patient who had intra-articular extension of the ischial osteotomy.[13,64] Intra-articular extension of the ischial osteotomy injures the acetabular branch of the obturator artery,[15] which may have led to the osteonecrosis seen in this patient. Intra-articular extension of an osteotomy cut is considered a technical complication and can also result in articular incongruity, nonunion, or loss of correction.[13,14] Nonunions have been reported in multiple series.[6,13,14,51,64] This is one reason for 6 to 8 weeks of limited weight bearing postoperatively, despite that many patients with ischial or pubic nonunions are asymptomatic. Other reported complications include wound

hematoma or infection,[51,64] venous thrombosis,[69] and heterotopic ossification.[6,13,51,86] The overall incidence of venous thrombosis is low, with a rate of 9.4 per 1000 in a multicenter series.[69] Reports of heterotopic ossification decreased dramatically once the abductors were routinely preserved. Finally, continued instability or impingement from either overcorrection or undercorrection has also been reported as a complication.[13] The incidence of complications has decreased with the evolution of the surgical technique, the recognition of FAI, and improvements in preoperative imaging and surgical planning.

SUMMARY

The Bernese PAO has now been performed for nearly 30 years. In that time, it has proved itself a technically complex procedure with the potential to considerably improve the natural history of the dysplastic hip. Significant refinements in the surgical technique combined with the recognition of FAI, improvements in the understanding of hip biomechanics and acetabular orientation, and more discerning patient selection have improved the outcomes related to this procedure. Although the recovery can be demanding and the potential for complications exists, the results are reproducible and the technique has become the gold standard for acetabular reorientation.

REFERENCES

1. Leunig M, Siebenrock KA, Ganz R. Instructional Course Lecture, American Academy of Orthopaedic Surgeons. Rationale of periacetabular osteotomy and background work. J Bone Joint Surg Am 2001;83:437–47.

2. Mechlenburg I, Nyengaard JR, Rømer L, et al. Changes in load-bearing area after Ganz periacetabular osteotomy evaluated by multislice CT scanning and stereology. Acta Orthop Scand 2004;75:147–53.

3. Maeyama A, Naito M, Moriyama S, et al. Periacetabular osteotomy reduces the dynamic instability of dysplastic hips. J Bone Joint Surg Br 2009;91:1438–42.

4. Rab GT. Lateral acetabular rotation improves anterior hip subluxation. Clin Orthop Relat Res 2007;456:170–5.

5. Ganz R, Klaue K, Vinh TS, et al. A new periacetabular osteotomy for the treatment of hip dysplasias. Clin Orthop Relat Res 1988;232:26–36.

6. Siebenrock KA, Leunig M, Ganz R. Instructional course lecture, american academy of orthopaedic surgeons. periacetabular osteotomy: the Bernese experience. J Bone Joint Surg Am 2001;83:449–55.

7. Loder RT, Karol LA, Johnson S. Influence of pelvic osteotomy on birth canal size. Arch Orthop Trauma Surg 1993;112:210–4.

8. Flückiger G, Eggli S, Kosina J, et al. Birth after Bernese periacetabular osteotomy. Geburt nach periazetabulärer Osteotomie. Orthopäde 2000;29:63–7 [in German].

9. Trousdale RT, Cabanela ME, Berry DJ, et al. Magnetic resonance imaging pelvimetry before and after periacetabular osteotomy. J Bone Joint Surg Am 2002;84:552–6.

10. Haddad FS, Garbuz DS, Duncan CP, et al. CT evaluation of periacetabular osteotomies. J Bone Joint Surg Br 2000;82:526–31.

11. Clohisy JC, Schutz AL, St. John L, et al. Periacetabular osteotomy. A systematic literature review. Clin Orthop Relat Res 2009;467:2041–52.

12. Clohisy JC, Barrett SE, Gordon JE, et al. Periacetabular osteotomy for the treatment of severe acetabular dysplasia. J Bone Joint Surg Am 2005;87:254–9.

13. Hussell JG, Rodriguez JA, Ganz R. Technical complications of the Bernese periacetabular osteotomy. Clin Orthop Relat Res 1999;363:81–92.

14. Peters CL, Erickson JA, Hines JL. Early results of the Bernese periacetabular osteotomy: the learning curve at an academic medical center. J Bone Joint Surg Am 2006;88:1920–6.

15. Beck M, Leunig M, Ellis T, et al. The acetabular blood supply: implications for periacetabular osteotomies. Surg Radiol Anat 2003;25:361–7.

16. Kalhor M, Beck M, Huff TW, et al. Capsular and pericapsular contributions to acetabular and femoral head perfusion. J Bone Joint Surg Am 2009;91:409–18.

17. Valenzuela RG, Cabanela ME, Trousdale RT. Sexual activity, pregnancy and childbirth after periacetabular osteotomy. Clin Orthop Relat Res 2004;418:146–52.

18. Leunig M, Ganz R. Bernese periacetabular osteotomy. Berner periazetabuläre Osteotomie. Orthopäde 1998;27:743–50 [in German].

19. Sucato DJ, Tulchin K, Shrader MW, et al. Gait, hip strength and functional outcomes after a Ganz periacetabular osteotomy for adolescent hip dysplasia. J Pediatr Orthop 2010;30:344–50.

20. Myers SR, Eijer H, Ganz R. Anterior femoroacetabular impingement after periacetabular osteotomy. Clin Orthop Relat Res 1999;363:93–9.

21. Steppacher SD, Tannast M, Werlen S, et al. Femoral morphology differs between deficient and excessive acetabular coverage. Clin Orthop Relat Res 2008;466:782–90.

22. Beck M, Woo A, Leunig M, et al. Gluteus minimus-induced femoral head deformation in dysplasia of the hip. Acta Orthop Scand 2001;72:13–7.

23. Ganz R, Parvizi J, Beck M, et al. Femoroacetabular impingement: A cause for osteoarthritis of the hip. Clin Orthop Relat Res 2003;417:112–20.

24. Hussell JG, Mast JW, Mayo KA, et al. A comparison of different surgical approaches for the periacetabular osteotomy. Clin Orthop Relat Res 1999;363:64–72.

25. Kim HT, Woo SH, Lee JS, et al. A dual anteroposterior approach to the Bernese periacetabular osteotomy. J Bone Joint Surg Br 2009;91:877–82.

26. Gautier E, Ganz K, Krügel N, et al. Anatomy of the medial femoral circumflex artery and its surgical implications. J Bone Joint Surg Br 2000;82:679–83.

27. Kühnel SP, Kalberer FA, Dora CF. Periacetabular osteotomy: validation of intraoperative fluoroscopic monitoring of acetabular orientation. Hip Int 2011;21:303–10.

28. Troelsen A, Elmengaard B, Søballe K. Comparison of the minimally invasive and ilioinguinal approaches for periacetabular osteotomy. Acta Orthop 2008;79:777–84.

29. Troelsen A, Elmengaard B, Søballe K. A new minimally invasive transsartorial approach for periacetabular osteotomy. J Bone Joint Surg Am 2008;90:493–8.

30. Ross JR, Zaltz I, Nepple JJ, et al. Arthroscopic disease classification and interventions as an adjunct in the treatment of acetabular dysplasia. Am J Sports Med 2011;39(Suppl 1):72S–8S.

31. Zhao X, Chosa E, Totoribe K, et al. Effect of periacetabular osteotomy for acetabular dysplasia clarified by three-dimensional finite element analysis. J Orthop Sci 2010;15:632–40.

32. Hipp JA, Sugano N, Millis MB, et al. Planning acetabular redirection osteotomies based on joint contact pressures. Clin Orthop Relat Res 1999;364:134–43.

33. Mechlenburg I, Nyengaard JR, Rømer L, et al. Prospective bone density changes after periacetabular osteotomy: a metholdological study. Int Orthop 2005;29:281–6.

34. Mechlenburg I, Kold S, Søballe K. No change detected by DEXA in bone mineral density after periacetabular osteotomy. Acta Orthop Belg 2009;75:761–6.

35. Nakamura Y, Naito M, Akiyoshi Y, et al. Acetabular cysts heal after successful periacetabular osteotomy. Clin Orthop Relat Res 2006;454:120–6.

36. Mechlenburg I, Nyengaard JR, Gelineck J, et al. Cartilage thickness in the hip measured by MRI and stereology before and after periacetabular osteotomy. Clin Orthop Relat Res 2010;468:1884–90.

37. Rasquinha BJ, Sayani J, Rudan JF, et al. Articular surface remodeling of the hip after periacetabular osteotomy. Int J Comput Assist Radiol Surg 2012;7:241–8.

38. Pedersen EN, Alkjær T, Søballe K, et al. Walking pattern in 9 women with hip dysplasia 18 months after periacetabular osteotomy. Acta Orthop 2006;77:203–8.

39. Fujii M, Nakashima Y, Noguchi Y, et al. Effect of intraarticular lesions on the outcome of periacetabular ostetomy patients with symptomatic hip dysplasia. J Bone Joint Surg Br 2011;93:1449–56.

40. Leunig M, Ganz R. Evolution of technique and indications for the Bernese periacetabular osteomy. Bull NYU Hosp Jt Dis 2011;69(Suppl 1):S42–6.

41. Ohzono K, Sakai T, Haraguchi K, et al. The Osaka experience. The "dome osteotomy" with and without labral resection. Das Osaka Konzept. Die "dome osteotomy" mit und ohne Labrum resektion. Orthopäde 1998;27:759–64 [in German].

42. Clohisy JC, Nunley RM, Curry MC, et al. Periacetabular osteotomy for the treatment of acetabular dysplasia associated with major aspherical femoral head deformities. J Bone Joint Surg Am 2007;89:1417–23.

43. MacDonald SJ, Hersche O, Ganz R. Periacetabular osteotomy in the treatment of neurogenic acetabular dysplasia. J Bone Joint Surg Br 1999;81:975–8.

44. Katz DA, Kim YJ, Millis MB. Periacetabular osteotomy in patients with Down's syndrome. J Bone Joint Surg Br 2005;87:544–7.

45. Sierra RJ, Schoeniger SR, Millis M, et al. Periacetabular osteotomy for containment of the nonarthritic dysplastic hip secondary to poliomyelitis. J Bone Joint Surg Am 2010;92:2917–23.

46. Siebenrock KA, Schoeniger R, Ganz R. Anterior femoroacetabular impingement due to acetabular retroversion. J Bone Joint Surg Am 2003;85:278–86.

47. Fujii M, Nakashima Y, Yamamoto T, et al. Acetabular retroversion in developmental dysplasia of the hip. J Bone Joint Surg Am 2010;92:895–903.

48. Akiyama M, Nakashima Y, Fujii M, et al. Femoral anteversion is correlated with acetabular version and coverage in Asian women with anterior and global deficient subgroups of hip dysplasia: a CT study. Skeletal Radiol 2012 Feb 13. [Epub ahead of print].

49. Paley D, Pfeil J. Principles of deformity correction around the knee. Orthopäde 2000;29(1):18–38.

50. Steppacher SD, Tannast M, Ganz R, et al. Mean 20-year follow-up of Bernese periacetabular osteotomy. Clin Orthop Relat Res 2008;466:1633–44.

51. Matheney T, Kim YJ, Zurakowski D, et al. Intermediate to long-term results following the Bernese periacetabular osteotomy and predictors of clinical outcome. J Bone Joint Surg Am 2009;91:2113–23.

52. Millis MB, Kain M, Sierra R, et al. Periacetabular osteotomy for acetabular dysplasia in patients older than 40 years. Clin Orthop Relat Res 2009;467:2228–34.

53. Trousdale RT, Ekkernkamp A, Ganz R, et al. Periacetabular and intertrochanteric osteotomy for the treatment of osteoarthritis in dysplastic hips. J Bone Joint Surg Am 1995;77-A:73–85.

54. Murphy S, Deshmukh R. Periacetabular osteotomy. Preoperative radiographic predictors of outcome. Clin Orthop Relat Res 2002;405:168–74.

55. Cunningham T, Jessel R, Zurakowski D, et al. Delayed gadolinium-enhanced magnetic resonance imaging of cartilage to predict early failure of Bernese periacetabular osteotomy for hip dysplasia. J Bone Joint Surg Am 2006;88:1540–8.

56. Sharifi E, Sharifi H, Morshed S, et al. Cost-effectiveness analysis of periacetabular osteotomy. J Bone Joint Surg Am 2008;90:1447–56.

57. Dora C, Zurbach J, Hersche O, et al. Pathomorphologic characteristics of posttraumatic acetabular dysplasia. J Orthop Trauma 2000;14:483–9.

58. Liporace FA, Ong B, Mohaideen A, et al. Development and injury of the triradiate cartilage with its effects on acetabular development: review of the literature. J Trauma 2003;54:1245–9.

59. Clohisy JC, Carlisle JC, Beaulé PE, et al. A systematic approach to the plain radiographic evaluation of the young adult hip. J Bone Joint Surg 2008;90(Suppl 4):47–66.

60. Potter HG, Black BR, Chong le R. New techniques in articular cartilage imaging. Clin Sports Med 2009;28:77–94.

61. Üzel M, Akkin SM, Tanyeli E, et al. Relationship of the lateral femoral cutaneous nerve to bony landmarks. Clin Orthop Relat Res 2011;469:2605–11.

62. Babst D, Steppacher SD, Ganz R, et al. The iliocapsularis muscle. An important stabilizer in the dysplastic hip. Clin Orthop Relat Res 2011;469:1728–34.

63. Pring ME, Trousdale RT, Cabanaela ME, et al. Intraoperative electromyographic monitoring during periacetabular surgery. Clin Orthop Relat Res 2002;400:158–64.

64. Thawrani D, Sucato DJ, Podeszwa DA, et al. Complications associated with the Bernese periacetabular osteotomy for hip dysplasia in adolescents. J Bone Joint Surg Am 2010;92:1707–14.

65. Shiramizu K, Naito M, Asayama I, et al. A quantitative anatomic characterization of the quadrilateral surface for periacetabular osteotomy. Clin Orthop Relat Res 2004;418:157–61.

66. Clohisy JC, Barrett SE, Gordon JE, et al. Periacetabular osteotomy in the treatment of severe acetabular dysplasia. Surgical Technique. J Bone Joint Surg Am 2006;88(Suppl 1):65–83.

67. Babis GC, Trousdale RT, Jenkyn TR, et al. Comparison of two methods of screw fixation in periacetabular osteotomy. Clin Orthop Relat Res 2002;403:221–7.

68. Widmer BJ, Peters CL, Bachus KN, et al. Initial stability of the acetabular fragment after periacetabular osteotomy: a biomechanical study. J Pediatr Orthop 2010;30:443–8.

69. Zaltz I, Beaulé P, Clohisy J, et al. Incidence of deep vein thrombosis and pulmonary embolus following periacetabular osteotomy. J Bone Joint Surg Am 2011;93(Suppl 2):62–5.

70. Hsieh PH, Huang KC, Lee PC, et al. Comparison of periacetabular osteotomy and total hip replacement in the same patient: a two- to ten-year follow-up study. J Bone Joint Surg Br 2009;91(7):883–8.

71. Parvizi J, Burmeister H, Ganz R. Previous Bernese periacetabular osteotomy does not compromise the results of total hip arthroplasty. Clin Orthop Relat Res 2004;423:118–22.

72. Troelsen A, Elmengaard B, Søballe K. Medium-term outcome of periacetabular osteotomy and predictors of conversion to total hip replacement. J Bone Joint Surg Am 2009;91(9):2169–79.

73. Murphy SB, Ganz R, Müller ME. The prognosis in untreated dysplasia of the hip. A study of radiographic factors that predict the outcome. J Bone Joint Surg Am 1995;77:985–9.

74. Polkowski GG, Novais EN, Kim YJ, et al. Does previous reconstructive surgery influence functional improvement and deformity correction after periacetabular osteotomy? Clin Orthop Relat Res 2012;470:516–24.

75. Teratani T, Naito M, Kiyama T, et al. Periacetabular osteotomy in patients fifty years of age or older. J Bone Joint Surg Am 2010;92:31–41.

76. Ito H, Tanino H, Yamanaka Y, et al. Intermediate to long-term results of periacetabular osteotomy in patients younger and older than forty years of age. J Bone Joint Surg Am 2011;93:1347–54.

77. Byrd JW, Jones KS. Hip arthroscopy in the presence of dysplasia. Arthroscopy 2003;19(10):1055–60.

78. Mei-Dan O, McConkey MO, Brick M. Catastrophic failure of hip arthroscopy due to iatrogenic instability: Can partial division of the ligamentum teres and iliofemoral ligament cause subluxation? Arthroscopy 2012;28:440–5.

79. Fujii M, Nakashima Y, Jingushi S, et al. Intraarticular findings in symptomatic developmental dysplasia of the hip. J Pediatr Orthop 2009;29(1):9–13.

80. Crawford MJ, Dy CJ, Alexander JW, et al. The biomechanics of the hip labrum and the stability of the hip. Clin Orthop Relat Res 2007;465:16–22.

81. Ferguson SJ, Bryant JT, Ganz R, et al. An in vitro investigation of the acetabular labral seal in hip joint mechanics. J Biomech 2003;36:171–8.

82. Ferguson SJ, Bryant JT, Ganz R, et al. The acetabular labrum seal: a poroelastic finite element model. Clin Biomech 2000;15:463–8.

83. Ferguson SJ, Bryant JT, Ganz R, et al. The influence of the acetabular labrum on hip joint cartilage consolidation: a poroelastic finite element model. J Biomech 2000;33:953–60.

84. Ferguson SJ, Bryant JT, Ito K. The material properties of the bovine acetabular labrum. J Orthop Res 2001;19:887–96.

85. Greaves LL, Gilbart MK, Yung AC, et al. Effect of acetabular labral tears, repair and resection on hip cartilage strain: a 7T MRI study. J Biomech 2010;43:858–63.

86. Myers CA, Register BC, Lertwanich P, et al. Role of the acetabular labrum and the iliofemoral ligament in hip stability. Am J Sports Med 2011;39(Suppl 1):85S–91S.

87. Ziebarth K, Balakumar J, Domayer S, et al. Bernese periacetabular osteotomy in males: is there an increased risk of femoroacetabular impingement (FAI) after Bernese periacetabular osteotomy? Clin Orthop Relat Res 2011;469(2):447–53.

Total Hip Arthroplasty and Hip Resurfacing Arthroplasty in the Very Young Patient

M. Wade Shrader, MD

KEYWORDS

• Hip • Arthroplasty • Resurfacing • Gait • Pediatrics

KEY POINTS

- Pediatric hip disorders can lead to early end-stage arthritis of the hip.
- Both total hip arthroplasty and hip resurfacing arthroplasty are options for the surgical treatment of hip arthritis in adolescents and young adults.
- Early reports comparing the 2 treatment options are difficult to interpret, and drawing definitive conclusions is difficult because they do not have sufficient evidence.
- Issues related to metal ions from metal-on-metal bearing surfaces should be considered.

INTRODUCTION

At present, hip arthroplasty is one of the most successful medical procedures available to the world, in terms of pain relief, return to function, and improvement in the quality of life for patients with hip arthritis. However, the success rate of total hip arthroplasty (THA) is noticeably lower in younger and more active patients.[1–4] Problems of prosthetic loosening, wear, osteolysis, and a shortening prosthetic life span have all been documented with higher frequency in younger patients.[5,6]

The indications for hip arthroplasty in the very young adult are the same as that in older patients: significant pain, decreased function, and a poor quality of life because of hip arthritis. However, because of the relatively higher risks involved with the longevity of the prosthesis, both patients and surgeons alike are cautious before proceeding to arthroplasty in such young patients. Furthermore, these surgical procedures are often technically demanding because of underlying severe deformity of both the femur and pelvis and previous surgery.

Although arthroplasty is never performed cavalierly in pediatric patients and very young adults (younger than 30 years), pathologic conditions may be so severe that arthroplasty or arthrodesis is the only viable option. At present, hip arthrodesis is less commonly performed because of advances in arthroplasty techniques and materials. Yet, at times, arthrodesis may be considered in the very young patient. The general thought is that hip arthrodesis gives a good outcome with a near normal gait pattern. However, there have been no studies that have investigated the functional activities of daily living, which most likely would be severely limited by hip arthrodesis. There are no contemporary series that discuss and compare hip arthrodesis to THA or hip resurfacing arthroplasty (HRA). An active patient does not often accept arthrodesis as a viable treatment option.

Even with the known difficulties, several series have reported great success with THA in young patients. Previous studies on the clinical outcome or cost-effectiveness of THA have objectively rated it as one of the most successful interventions in modern day medicine. Uncemented

Division of Pediatric Orthopaedic Surgery, Phoenix Children's Hospital, 1919 East Thomas Road, Phoenix, AZ 85016, USA
E-mail address: mwshrader@phoenixchildrens.com

Orthop Clin N Am 43 (2012) 359–367
doi:10.1016/j.ocl.2012.05.005

orthopedic.theclinics.com

components are the mainstay in most arthroplasty cases today, and clinical results have shown excellent longevity, with a 10-year survivorship of more than 95% documented in multiple reports.[1–6]

HRA has recently been reintroduced as a possible alternative for young active patients with hip arthritis. Original reports from the developers of some of the newer HRA systems have shown excellent midterm results, with a 10-year survivorship of 98%.[7–9] Furthermore, motion analysis laboratory studies have suggested more normal function for patients receiving HRA in comparison with patients receiving traditional THA.[10,11] However, recent reports, in the national joint registries, of higher failure rates in some HRA systems have tempered some of the initial excitement for HRA.[12–14] The higher revision rates coupled with concerns about metal ions, metal hypersensitivity reactions, and pseudotumors have thrown the future of resurfacing into ambiguity.[15–17] One of the main criticisms of HRA is that it is much more technically demanding than THA, with a significantly steep learning curve.[18,19] Nevertheless, many investigators maintain that HRA is an excellent treatment option for the very active and very young patient with end-stage hip disease.[20]

The purpose of this article is to discuss end-stage hip pathologic conditions in pediatric and adolescent patients and the pros and cons of THA and HRA in adolescents and the very young adult and to put forward special issues that should be considered when treating these young patients.

ETIOLOGY OF HIP ARTHRITIS IN PEDIATRIC PATIENTS AND YOUNG ADULTS

Hip arthritis is relatively rare in pediatric patients, adolescents, and adults younger than 40 years. However, several pathologic conditions predispose certain patients to have a higher risk of joint deterioration than the general population. Most experts in adult hip arthritis believe that osteoarthritis of the hip in adults mainly occurs from a more definitive specific pathologic condition that is responsible for the arthritis. Some of the more common pathologies encountered in the very young adult patient include developmental dysplasia of the hip (DDH), femoral acetabular impingement (FAI), Perthes disease, slipped capital femoral epiphysis (SCFE), avascular necrosis (AVN), and inflammatory arthritis. (Please note: THA and DDH, FAI, AVN, and inflammatory arthritis have been discussed elsewhere in this issue, and the technical details of surgical technique for these pathologic conditions are not discussed in this article.)[21,22]

DDH

From infancy to adulthood, DDH describes a wide spectrum of pathologic conditions in which the hip joint itself has abnormal morphology that leads to pain and dysfunction and ultimately, in many cases, joint replacement (**Fig. 1**).[23,24] Newborn screening and early treatment strategies, such as the Pavlik harness, have reduced the cases of untreated hip dysplasia. In cases of hip dysplasia that go undetected in newborn screening or are resistant to harness therapy, treatment with closed/open reduction and pelvic osteotomies is effective in reducing the long-term sequelae of DDH.[25] The advent of periacetabular osteotomy has improved nonarthroplasty outcomes in the patient with symptomatic DDH in adolescence and young adulthood.[26–28] The long-term outcome of severe and undertreated DDH is significant hip arthritis for which the appropriate treatment is arthroplasty.[29,30]

Very young patients with neuromuscular hip dysplasia may progress sooner to end-stage hip arthritis than to DDH. Patients with cerebral palsy, Down syndrome, and other neuromuscular diseases often have severe hip dysplasia. Hip arthroplasty carries a high risk of complications in these disorders, including instability, infection, and loosening. Yet in the carefully selected patient, arthroplasty may be a solution to give these patients a better quality of life (**Fig. 2**).

FAI

Advances in the knowledge of hip pathophysiology have increased the understanding of how FAI leads to hip arthritis.[31] In the pediatric patient, FAI can occur from several primary pathologic conditions, such as Perthes disease or SCFE. Idiopathic FAI results from 2 primary mechanisms: cam and pincer impingement. If left untreated, FAI can lead to cartilage delamination, overloading of the joint cartilage, and, ultimately, end-stage arthritis. Young adults with FAI now have effective treatment options in the form of surgical hip dislocation and femoral head osteoplasty, which can safely improve the biomechanics of the joint with low risks of iatrogenic AVN.[32–35]

PERTHES DISEASE

Perthes disease is a poorly understood disorder that is associated with a disruption of the blood supply to the growing femoral head in children. The characteristic sequence of epiphyseal growth retardation, sclerosis, fragmentation, and reossification leads to coxa magna and both

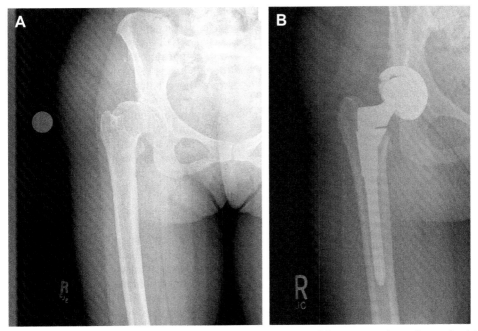

Fig. 1. (*A*) Preoperative radiograph of an 18-year-old woman with DDH. (*B*) Postoperative radiograph with uncemented THA.

femoral and acetabular deformity, which often becomes symptomatic in adolescence and young adulthood.[36] The efficacy of surgical treatment in the pediatric patient is still under debate.[37,38] Adults with early onset symptoms may benefit from FAI treatment techniques. Severe deformity results in the need for arthroplasty in early adulthood.[39]

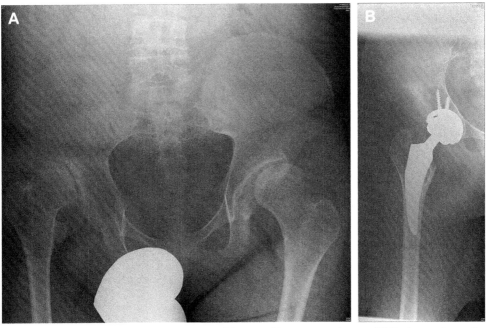

Fig. 2. (*A*) Preoperative radiograph of an 18-year old man with Down syndrome. (*B*) Postoperative radiograph with uncemented THA.

SCFE

Many factors are thought to contribute to the pathophysiology of SCFE, including body habitus and adolescent obesity, hormonal disorders, and mechanical factors.[40] The incidence varies widely across different regions, and this regional variation is largely unexplained.[41] In situ pinning has been the mainstay for the treatment of children with SCFE, and for mild to moderate cases, this treatment seems to stabilize the deformity and lead to relatively normal hip function.[42] However, patients with more severe slips and those who progress on to AVN develop early osteoarthritis requiring arthroplasty.[43] As in other areas of hip pathology in the adolescent and young adult, newer treatment options have been designed with the aim of increasing the longevity of these slipped hips. Acute surgical hip dislocation and open reduction of SCFE have been reported in small series, which have resulted in excellent resolution of the deformity seemingly without an increase in the progression to AVN from the baseline risk that SCFE naturally brings.[44,45] FAI techniques can also be used in the chronic setting, with the goal being to decrease impingement that leads to chondral damage and hip arthritis.

AVN

AVN, also known as osteonecrosis, of the hip comes from a wide range of primary pathologic conditions.[46] AVN typically affects young adults aged 30 to 40 years but can affect pediatric patients in their teenage years. Exposure to several risk factors can lead to AVN, including sickle cell disease, thrombophilia, use of alcohol and corticosteroids, and myeloproliferative disorders, such as leukemia or Gaucher disease. AVN from these latter disorders can come from the disease process itself or the treatments, such as chemotherapy and chronic use of steroids. Early stages of AVN can be effectively treated with non-arthroplasty techniques, such as core decompression or vascularized free fibular implantation. Larger lesions and more advanced collapse can only be effectively treated with arthoplasty.[47]

OTHERS

The most common pathologic conditions causing end-stage hip disease in an adolescent or young adult have been discussed earlier. However, there are several other disease processes that can also destroy the hip joint, necessitating arthroplasty. Inflammatory arthropathies, including rheumatoid arthritis and ankylosing spondylitis, can lead to hip pathologic conditions requiring arthroplasty at a young age.[48] Idiopathic chondrolysis can cause rapid destruction of the hip cartilage without a specific known causative factor. Posttraumatic arthritis can occur after high-energy trauma, such as hip dislocation, acetabular fractures, or femoral head fractures (**Fig. 3**). Infections can also cause significant destruction of the cartilage. A previously neglected or undertreated septic arthritis can leave children with a severely pathologic hip joint for the remainder of their life (**Fig. 4**).

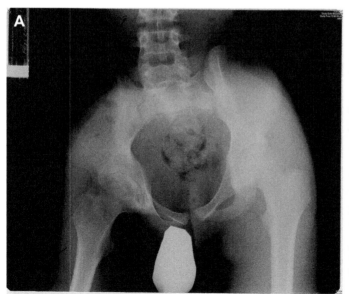
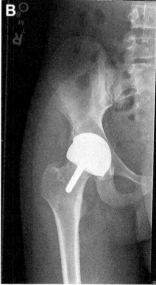

Fig. 3. (A) Preoperative radiograph of a 14-year-old man with end-stage hip arthritis after traumatic hip dislocation caused during bicycle motocross racing. (B) Postoperative radiograph after HRA.

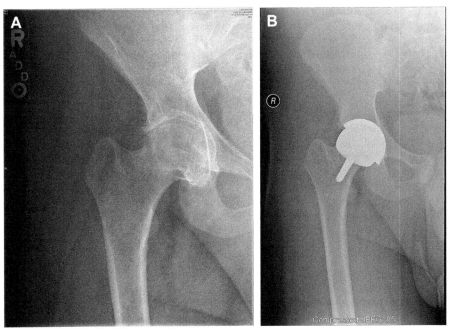

Fig. 4. (*A*) Preoperative radiograph of a 15-year-old man who had septic arthritis after hip arthroscopy for labral repair. (*B*) Postoperative radiograph after HRA.

CONSIDERATIONS OF THA VERSUS HRA IN YOUNG PATIENTS

The indications for both THA and HRA are similar: end-stage hip arthritis unresponsive to conservative treatment.[49,50] However, the technical differences between the 2 procedures make ideal patient selection, especially in the case of HRA, even more critical. HRA is indicated mostly for osteoarthritis or posttraumatic arthritis in the young male patient.[9,51] HRA may also be considered for cases of AVN without cysts larger than 1 cm and those with moderate deformity due to pediatric hip pathologic conditions.

SPECIFIC INDICATIONS

Many of the young patients being considered for HRA have coxarthrosis as a result of pediatric hip disease, including severe cases of SCFE, DDH, and Perthes disease. The relative benefits of HRA versus THA should be considered in each case. While many of these patients are young and of the ideal age to be a candidate for HRA, the altered anatomy of their primary disorders may make THA more effective in restoring optimal hip biomechanics.

Severe pelvic defects that are caused by DDH can make HRA more difficult if there is not enough acetabular bone stock to allow initial secure fixation of the monoblock resurfacing cup because that precludes the use of additional screw fixation. There are dysplasia cups in some of the HRA product lines.[52] These cups use peripheral screw fixation to supplement the press fit of the monoblock cup. However, there are very few reports on the efficacy of these cups, and, in general, HRA is contraindicated in cases of severe dysplasia (Crowe III and higher).

Patients with significant limb length inequality can benefit from an increased limb length, which can restore more normal gait with THA. Significant limb length differences cannot be addressed with HRA. This also means that the risk of an unwanted postoperative limb length inequality (a significant medical-legal issue) from HRA is much lesser than that from THA.

Coxarthrosis from disorders like SCFE, Perthes disease, and severe cam-type FAI can result in significant deformities of the femoral head and neck. HRA is predicated on resurfacing the femoral head without causing any damage to the femoral neck. Any damage to the neck during the preparation of the femoral component can lead to a high risk of failure due to postoperative femoral neck fracture. Patients with severe SCFE can exhibit a significant deviation in the femoral head in comparison with the femoral neck, which makes HRA even more technically challenging. A short wide femoral neck, as in the case of patients with severe Perthes disease, would also be a relative contraindication to HRA. A severe deformity caused by Perthes disease may make it difficult to achieve reliable fixation of the femoral component while avoiding extra-articular impingement.[39]

HRA can be performed in cases of AVN with small focal defects.[53] However, when HRA is performed in the setting of large AVN defects or significant femoral collapse, it can lead to early femoral component failures. HRA is contraindicated in patients with inadequate bone stock in the femoral head or neck. Patients with severe osteoporosis or those with large cysts in the femoral head-neck junction are at an unacceptably high risk for femoral neck fracture when HRA is performed. Patients with femoral neck lesions from any type of neoplasm or infection should also likely be treated with THA.

METAL IONS

The improvement in metallurgy has been one of the scientific advances that have allowed the resurgence of HRA. Metal-on-metal (MoM) HRA has shown much better clinical effectiveness than the early results of HRA with other materials. Similarly, MoM THA has been very popular in recent years both in the United States and abroad. Early studies in modern MoM-bearing surfaces did not show significant risks from metal ion absorption in patients who underwent those arthroplasties.

However, recent reports of some MoM implants have caused significant concerns. The potential for local soft tissue and systemic reactions to MoM ions is much higher with HRA than with THA.[15–17] The specific causes and the incidence of these adverse reactions in MoM HRA and THA remain incompletely understood. Any patient with known metal sensitivity should not receive an HRA or a MoM THA. Furthermore, women of childbearing age and potential should also not receive an HRA or a MoM THA because of the placental transfer of ions and potential issues with the development of the fetus.

A localized metal hypersensitivity, or pseudotumor formation, has also recently been described in MoM hip arthroplasties, both in MoM THA and MoM HRA.[17] Although the exact pathophysiology is not completely understood, it is thought that a local hypersensitivity reaction forms an aggressive response, which leads to soft tissue mass formation, possible osteolysis, prosthetic loosening, chronic severe pain, and ultimate failure of the implant.

REVISION RATES

One of the advantages of HRA is the concept of bone conservation; by not resecting the femoral head, by definition, HRA conserves more bone on the femoral side for later revisions. However, there has been some suggestion that the implant requirements of femur-acetabulum matching causes additional reaming on the pelvic side for HRA, usually in the order of 2 mm, resulting in the use of a larger cup than would have been used in traditional THA.

Bone conservation becomes a very important consideration when dealing with such young patients who may be facing more than 1 revision. Proponents of HRA argue that revision to THA is easier with resurfacing, allowing the surgeon to use a primary femoral stem rather than a revision-type stem. Furthermore, if the cup is well fixed in HRA, a femoral-only revision could be considered using a large head MoM femoral stem that is compatible. However, till date, there have been no studies that have documented easier revisions from HRA than from THA.

In the early series from Birmingham, HRA is very favorably compared to other THA series in young adults. The Birmingham Hip Resurfacing series have shown a survivorship of 98% at 10-year follow-up. This is similar in many aspects to multiple reports of uncemented THA. However, data from other HRA implants have shown significantly higher revision rates. There has been some suggestion that specific metallurgy techniques for a hip resurfacing and MoM device may be the reasons for the early failure of some systems.[54] The Australian Joint registry has also shown slightly higher rates of revision for some HRA systems in comparison with THA.[12] However, when isolated to very young patients, the HRA revision rate in the Australian registry is slightly lower than that for THA. Other national joint registries have also shown slightly higher revision rates for HRA in comparison with THA.[13,14] However, subgroup analyses for any of these databases should be considered and interpreted with caution.[55] There are yet to be conclusive high-level studies with appropriately matched patients that can help direct definitive conclusions about revision rates of HRA in comparison with THA.

These recent concerns have led the American Academy of Orthopaedic Surgeons and the Food and Drug Administration to issue a warning about HRA and MoM THA to the general public, warning them of certain implants that seem to have a revision rate that is higher than expected and cautioning patients who have symptoms of potential implant failure to seek immediate evaluation. Clearly, the future of MoM implants, in general, and the future of HRA, in particular, hinges on whether these revision rates are shown to be true across the spectrum of all implant systems and for comparable patient groups. The answer to that question should be evident in the next 5 to 10 years.

FUNCTIONAL RESULTS

An argument made by proponents of HRA is that many patients seem to claim that their hip feels "more normal" than when treated with THA. Because the question of HRA versus THA is considered in the young active patient, the ability to have a more functional lifestyle after hip arthroplasty is an important consideration. With improvement in implant technologies and excellent results in THA series, hip arthroplasty, both THA and HRA, is being considered in younger patients. Many of these young patients are not content accepting a pain-free hip while significantly altering their lifestyle. Indeed, many patients want a hip arthroplasty performed so they can continue to be active in a variety of challenging activities. The impact of these activities on the longevity of hip arthroplasties is yet to be determined. Nevertheless, expectations of higher activity levels are clearly becoming more common in younger patients.

There have been several studies that have documented differences in gait and functional activities after THA and HRA. Mont and colleagues[11] showed more normal hip kinematics at 1 year in patients treated with HRA than with THA. These findings were confirmed in a study that showed more normal hip moments in patients treated with HRA in comparison with patients treated with a relatively large head THA series.[10]

The mechanism for these more normal hip mechanics is uncertain. Each of these series could have confounding results with patient selection bias favoring the HRA results. HRA could produce a more physiologic loading of the proximal femur through the neck. The larger head size in both HRA and large head MoM THA could approximate the center of hip rotation better than the traditional THA. Differences in proprioception could provide a neuromuscular adaptation explanation for the differences found in these studies.

The determination of whether HRA truly provides better and more normal function is important, along with more definitive analysis of revision rates of HRA compared with similarly age-matched and demand-matched cohorts of THA. Better understanding of these 2 factors will go a long way toward determining the future of HRA.

SUMMARY

Severe hip arthritis in an adolescent or very young adult can be a devastating disability that affects all aspects of a patient's life. Newer treatment strategies in pediatric orthopedic surgery and hip preservation potentially could lessen the impact of this severe disorder in the future. Careful patient selection can lead to excellent outcomes for both THA and/or HRA in young patients. Further study will likely shed more light on whether HRA truly has more improved functional results than THA, and studies with longer follow-up that show definitive revision rates also should affect the future of HRA.

REFERENCES

1. Berry DJ, Cabanela ME. Primary uncemented total hip arthroplasty in patients less than 40 years of age [abstract]. Orthop Trans 1993–1994;17:588.
2. Callaghan JJ. Results of primary total hip arthroplasty in young patients. J Bone Joint Surg Am 1993;75:1728.
3. Clohisy JC, Oryhon JM, Seyler TM, et al. Function and fixation of total hip arthroplasty in patients 25 years of age or younger. Clin Orthop Relat Res 2010;468:3207–13.
4. Restrepo C, Lettich T, Roberts N, et al. Uncemented total hip arthroplasty in patients less than twenty-years. Acta Orthop Belg 2008;75(5):615–22.
5. Berry DJ, Torchia ME, Klassen RA. The young patient. In: Morrey BF, editor. Joint replacement arthroplasty. 2nd edition. New York: Churchill Livingstone; 1996. p. 1027.
6. Klassen RA, Parlasca RJ, Bianco AJ. Total joint arthroplasty: applications in children and adolescents. Mayo Clin Proc 1979;54:579.
7. Amstutz HC, Le Duff MJ. Eleven years of experience with metal-on-metal hybrid hip resurfacing: a review of 1000 conserve plus. J Arthroplasty 2008; 23(6 Suppl 1):36–43.
8. Treacy RB, McBryde CW, Shears E, et al. Birmingham hip resurfacing: a minimum follow-up of ten years. J Bone Joint Surg Br 2011;93(1):27–33.
9. Daniel J, Pynsent PB, McMinn DJ. Metal-on-metal resurfacing of the hip in patients under the age of 55 years with osteoarthritis. J Bone Joint Surg Br 2004;86(2):177–84.
10. Shrader MW, Bhowmik-Stoker M, Jacofsky MC, et al. Gait and stair function in total and resurfacing hip arthroplasty: a pilot study. Clin Orthop Relat Res 2009; 467(6):1476–84.
11. Mont MA, Seyler TM, Ragland PS, et al. Gait analysis of patients with resurfacing hip arthroplasty compared with hip osteoarthritis and standard total hip arthroplasty. J Arthroplasty 2007;22(1):100–8.
12. Australian Orthopaedic Association. National joint replacement registry. Annual report 2008. Adelaide (Australia): Australian Orthopaedic Association; 2008.

13. Karrholm J, Garrelick G, Rogmark C, et al. Swedish hip arthroplasty register. Annual report 2007 (English). Gothenburg (Sweden): Department of Orthopaedics, Sahlgrenska University Hospital; 2008.

14. National Joint Registry for England and Wales. 5th annual report. Hemel Hempstead (United Kingdom): National Joint Registry Center; 2009.

15. McGrory B, Barrack R, Lachiewicz P, et al. Modern metal-on-metal hip resurfacing. J Am Acad Orthop Surg 2010;18:306–14.

16. Vail TP. Hip resurfacing. J Am Acad Orthop Surg 2011;19:236–41.

17. Pandit H, Glyn-Jones S, McLardy-Smith P, et al. Pseudotumours associated with metal-on-metal hip resurfacings. J Bone Joint Surg Br 2008;90(7):847–51.

18. Della Valle CJ, Nunley RM, Raterman SJ, et al. Initial American experience with hip resurfacing following FDA approval. Clin Orthop Relat Res 2009;467(1):72–8.

19. Stulberg BN, Trier KK, Naughton M, et al. Results and lessons learned from a United States hip resurfacing investigational device exemption trial. J Bone Joint Surg Am 2009;90(Suppl 3):21–6.

20. Shimmin A, Beaulé PE, Campbell P. Metal-on-metal hip resurfacing arthroplasty. J Bone Joint Surg Am 2008;90(3):637–54.

21. Kim YJ. Residual pediatric hip deformities and their impact on the adult hip. In: Beaulé PE, Amadio PC, editors. The young adult with hip pain. Rosemont (IL): American Academy of Orthopaedic Surgeons; 2007. p. 21–36.

22. Schoenecker PL, Clohisy JC, Millis MB, et al. Surgical management of the problematic hip in adolescent and young adult patients. J Am Acad Orthop Surg 2011;19:275–86.

23. Weinstein SL, Mubarak SJ, Wenger DR. Developmental hip dysplasia and dislocation: part I. Instr Course Lect 2004;53:523–30.

24. Weinstein SL, Mubarak SJ, Wenger DR. Developmental hip dysplasia and dislocation: part II. Instr Course Lect 2004;53:531–42.

25. Mladenov K, Dora C, Wicart P, et al. Natural history of hips with borderline acetabular index and acetabular dysplasia in infants. J Pediatr Orthop 2002;22:607–12.

26. Ganz RH, Klaue K, Vinh TS, et al. A new periacetabular osteotomy for the treatment of hip dysplasias. Technique and preliminary results. Clin Orthop 1988;232:26.

27. Kim YJ, Ganz R, Murphy SB, et al. Hip joint-preserving surgery: beyond the classic osteotomy. Instr Course Lect 2006;55:145–58.

28. Steppacher SD, Tannast M, Ganz R, et al. Mean 20-year follow-up Bernese periacetabular osteotomy. Clin Orthop Relat Res 2008;466(7):1633–44.

29. Albinana J, Dolan LA, Spratt KF, et al. Acetabular dysplasia after treatment for developmental dysplasia

of the hip: implications for secondary procedures. J Bone Joint Surg Br 2004;86:876–86.

30. Luhmann SJ, Bassett GS, Gordon JR, et al. Reduction of a dislocation of the hip due to developmental dysplasia: implications for the need for future surgery. J Bone Joint Surg Am 2003;85:239–43.

31. Parvizi J, Leunig M, Ganz R. Femoroacetabular impingement. J Am Acad Orthop Surg 2007;15(9):561–70.

32. Ganz R, Gill TJ, Gautier E, et al. Surgical dislocation of the adult hip: a technique with full access to the femoral head and acetabulum without the risk of avascular necrosis. J Bone Joint Surg Br 2001;83(8):1119–24.

33. Sierra RJ, Trousdale RT, Ganz R, et al. Hip disease in the young active patient: evaluation and nonarthroplasty surgical options. J Am Acad Orthop Surg 2008;16(12):689–703.

34. Beaulé PE, Allen DJ, Clohisy JC, et al. The young adult with hip impingement: deciding on the optimal intervention. J Bone Joint Surg Am 2009;91(1):210–21.

35. Clohisy JC, Zebala LP, Nepple JJ, et al. Combined hip arthroscopy and limited open osteochondroplasty for anterior femoroacetabular impingement. J Bone Joint Surg Am 2010;92(8):1697–706.

36. Catterall A. The natural history of Perthes' disease. J Bone Joint Surg Br 1971;53:37–53.

37. Herring J, Hui K, Browne R. Legg-Calvé-Perthes disease. Part I: classification of radiographs with use of the modified lateral pillar and Stulberg classifications. J Bone Joint Surg Am 2004;86(10):2103–20.

38. Herring J, Hui K, Browne R. Legg-Calvé-Perthes disease. Part II: prospective multicenter study of the effect of the treatment on outcome. J Bone Joint Surg Am 2004;86(10):2121–33.

39. Costa CR, Johnson AJ, Naziri Q, et al. Review of total hip resurfacing and total hip arthroplasty in young patients who had Legg-Calvé-Perthes disease. Orthop Clin North Am 2011;42(3):419–22.

40. Loder RT, Aronsson DD, Weinstein SL, et al. Slipped capital femoral epiphysis. Instr Course Lect 2008;57:473–98.

41. Loder RT, Starnes T, Dikos G, et al. Demographic predictors of severity of stable slipped capital femoral epiphyses. J Bone Joint Surg Am 2006;88(1):97–105.

42. Carney BT, Weinstein SL, Noble J. Long-term follow-up of slipped capital femoral epiphysis. J Bone Joint Surg 1991;73:667–74.

43. Kennedy JG, Hresko MT, Kasser JR, et al. Osteonecrosis of the femoral head associated with slipped capital femoral epiphysis. J Pediatr Orthop 2001;21(2):189–93.

44. Leunig M, Slongo T, Ganz R. Subcapital realignment in slipped capital femoral epiphysis: surgical hip

dislocation and trimming of the stable trochanter to protect the perfusion of the epiphysis. Instr Course Lect 2008;57:499–507.

45. Chen RC, Schoenecker PL, Dobbs MB, et al. Urgent reduction, fixation, and arthrotomy for unstable slipped capital femoral epiphysis. J Pediatr Orthop 2009;297(7):687–94.

46. Urbaniak JR, Jones JP Jr, editors. Osteonecrosis: etiology, diagnosis and treatment. Rosemont (IL): American Academy of Orthop Surg; 1997.

47. Mont MA, Hungerford DS. Non-traumatic avascular necrosis of the femoral head. J Bone Joint Surg Am 1995;77:459–74.

48. Arden GP, Ansell BM, Hunter MJ. Total hip replacement in juvenile chronic polyarthritis and ankylosing spondylitis. Clin Orthop 1972;84:130.

49. Mont MA, Maar DC, Krackow KA, et al. Total hip replacement without cement for non-inflammatory osteoarthrosis in patients who are less than forty-five years old. J Bone Joint Surg Am 1993;75:740.

50. Pollard TC, Baker RP, Eastaugh-Waring SJ, et al. Treatment of the young active patient with osteoarthritis of the hip. A five- to seven-year comparison of hybrid total hip arthroplasty and metal-on-metal resurfacing. J Bone Joint Surg Br 2006;88(5):592–600.

51. Johnson AJ, Zywiel MG, Maduekwe UI, et al. Is resurfacing arthroplasty appropriate for posttraumatic osteoarthritis? Clin Orthop Relat Res 2011;469(6):1567–73.

52. McMinn DJ, Daniel J, Ziaee H, et al. Results of the Birmingham Hip Resurfacing dysplasia component in severe acetabular insufficiency: a six-to 9.6-year follow-up. J Bone Joint Surg Br 2008;90(6):715–23.

53. Sayeed SA, Johnson AJ, Stroh DA, et al. Hip resurfacing in patients who have osteonecrosis and are 25 years or under. Clin Orthop Relat Res 2011;469(6):1582–8.

54. Daniel J, Ziaee H, Kamali A, et al. Ten-year results of a double-heat-treated metal-on-metal hip resurfacing. J Bone Joint Surg Br 2010;92(1):20–7.

55. Corten K, MacDonald SJ. Hip resurfacing data from national joint registries: what do they tell us? What do they not tell us? Clin Orthop Relat Res 2010;468(2):351–7.

Acetabular Considerations During Total Hip Arthroplasty for Hip Dysplasia

Michele R. Dapuzzo, MD[a], Rafael J. Sierra, MD[b],*

KEYWORDS

- Developmental dysplasia of the hip (DDH) • Total hip arthroplasty (THA) • Femoral head autograft
- Acetabular reconstruction • Uncemented acetabulum

KEY POINTS

- The wide spectrum of anatomic abnormalities that characterize hip dysplasia dictate the need for different reconstructive techniques when hip replacement is required.
- When standard techniques of reconstruction leave a significant portion of the component uncovered, the alternatives include acetabular augmentation with bone autograft, intentional high placement of the component, or medialization of the component with or without medial wall osteotomy.
- Uncemented sockets have provided promising midterm results with supplemental bone augmentation and are our preferred method of treatment for hips with moderate dysplasia and anterolateral acetabular bone deficiency.

INTRODUCTION

Developmental dysplasia of the hip (DDH) is the most prevalent developmental childhood hip disorder.[1] Formerly known as congenital dysplasia of the hip, this condition encompasses abnormalities involving the growing hip, from minimal dysplasia to dislocation of the hip joint. Dysplastic hips share a common pathophysiology in which anatomic abnormalities subject the hip to increased contact stress leading to abnormal hip biomechanics, hip instability, impingement, associated labral pathologic condition, and eventually degenerative arthritis.[2–4] Despite the availability of several nonarthroplastic alternatives, many patients with advanced hip dysplasia eventually require hip replacement surgery. Because of the unique characteristics of these patients, including young age and anatomic abnormalities of the hip, the failure rate after total hip arthroplasty (THA) in patients with DDH is higher than those in the general population.[5] The specific alterations observed in the acetabulum usually include a shallow socket with bone deficiency anteriorly, laterally, and superiorly. Reconstruction during THA, particularly the location of the placement of the acetabular component defines the new center of hip rotation, which in turn influences hip biomechanics, leg length, and femoral reconstruction. This article reviews the different alternatives for the reconstruction of acetabulum during THA in patients with DDH.

CLASSIFICATION

Dysplastic hips can be characterized by the severity of anatomic abnormalities. Classification systems are useful for the assessment of patients and comparison of results using different treatments. The classification by Crowe and colleagues[6] is the most common method to categorize the degree of dysplasia. In the original

[a] Department of Orthopaedic Surgery, University of Virginia, PO Box 800159, Charlottesville, VA 22908, USA;
[b] Department of Orthopedic Surgery, Mayo Clinic, 200 First Street Southwest, Rochester, MN 55905, USA
* Corresponding author.
E-mail address: Sierra.Rafael@mayo.edu

Orthop Clin N Am 43 (2012) 369–375
doi:10.1016/j.ocl.2012.05.012
0030-5898/12/$ – see front matter © 2012 Elsevier Inc. All rights reserved.

description, dysplastic hips were categorized radiographically into 4 groups based on the extent of proximal migration of the femoral head. The migration is calculated on an anteroposterior radiograph of the pelvis by measuring the vertical distance between the interteardrop line and the inferior head-neck junction. The amount of subluxation is the ratio between this distance and the vertical diameter of the undeformed femoral head. Thus, if the distance between the head-neck junction and the teardrop is half the vertical diameter of the femoral head, the hip is subluxated 50%. When the femoral head is deformed, the predicted vertical diameter of the femoral head was 20% of the height of the pelvis, as measured from the highest point on the iliac crest to the inferior margin of the ischial tuberosity (**Table 1**). Because this system is based on the degree of displacement of the femoral head and does not define the acetabular abnormality, other classification systems, such as the Hartofilakidis classification,[7] which divides congenital hip disease in adults into 3 categories: dysplasia, low dislocation, and high dislocation (**Table 2**), have been proposed. The authors prefer using this classification system because it simply describes the acetabular deformity and is useful in determining the type of acetabular reconstruction that is required. In this system, each category is based on the relationship between the femoral head and the true or false acetabulum. With dysplasia, the femoral head, despite some degree of subluxation, is still contained within the original acetabulum. With low dislocation, the femoral head articulates with a false acetabulum that partially covers the true acetabulum and radiographically appears to be 2 overlapping acetabula; the inferior part of the false acetabulum is an osteophyte that begins at the level of the superior rim of the true acetabulum. With high dislocation, the femoral head migrates superiorly and posteriorly. The true acetabulum is inferior and anterior to the hollow in the iliac wing, with which the femoral head articulates, and may have the appearance of a false acetabulum.

ANATOMIC POSITION OF THE ACETABULAR COMPONENT

To reconstruct the acetabulum successfully during THA in patients with DDH, certain information such as the position of the true acetabulum is of capital importance. Today, the aim of the acetabular reconstruction is to place the acetabular component in the area of the true acetabulum for purely mechanical reasons. A method to locate the correct anatomic position of the acetabulum in deformed hips and to assess any variation of position of the acetabular component after THA based on radiographs was developed by Ranawat and colleagues.[8] Parallel horizontal lines are drawn at the level of the iliac crest and the ischial tuberosities and are connected by a perpendicular passing through a point (A) located 5 mm lateral to the intersection of Kohler and Shenton lines. The length of the perpendicular between the parallels lines is equal to the height of the pelvis and one-fifth of this equals the height of the acetabulum. A second point (B) is located on the perpendicular superior to the point A, at a distance equal to one-fifth of the perpendicular line. From B a perpendicular is erected laterally to point C, so that the distance BC equals the distance AB. Joining point A and C completes the isosceles triangle, indicating the correct position of the acetabulum to be reconstructed. In a normal hip, the superior border of the triangle will pass through the superior aspect of the subchondral bone of the acetabulum (**Fig. 1**). Although this system is useful, in the majority of deformed hips, the location of the radiographic teardrop is visible and can be used as a simple radiographic marker to the position of the acetabular component.

TREATMENT OPTIONS

When choosing a treatment option for acetabular reconstruction, risk and benefits of the technique as well as the type of bony deformity should be considered preoperatively. The practical and biomechanical advantages of hip reconstruction at a normal anatomic location must be balanced with the need to provide sufficient acetabular implant coverage. When possible, acetabular reconstruction should seek normalization of the

Table 1	
Crowe classification for DDH in adults	
Group	**Description**
I	Subluxation <50% or proximal dislocation <0.1% of the pelvic height <10%
II	Subluxation 50%–75% or proximal dislocation of 0.1%–0.15% of pelvic height 10%–15%
III	Subluxation 75%–100% or proximal dislocation of 0.15%–0.20% of pelvic height 15%–20%
IV	Subluxation >100% or proximal dislocation of >0.20% of pelvic height >20%

Table 2
The Hartofilakidis classification for DDH in adults

Type	Description	Acetabular Deficiencies During Surgery
Dysplastic hip	The femoral head is contained within the original acetabulum despite the degree of subluxation	• Segmental deficiency of the superior wall • Secondary shallowness due to fossa-covering osteophyte
Low dislocation	The femoral head articulates with a false acetabulum that partially covers the true acetabulum to a varying degree	• Complete absence of the superior wall • Anterior and posterior segmental deficiency • Narrow opening and inadequate depth of the true acetabulum
High dislocation	The femoral head is completely out of the true acetabulum and migrated superiorly and posteriorly to a varying degree	• Segmental deficiency of the entire with narrow opening • Inadequate depth • Excessive anteversion • Abnormal distribution of bone stock, mainly located superoposteriorly in relation to the true acetabulum

hip center of rotation.[9] Because of the anatomic abnormalities, placement of standard-sized acetabular components in a dysplastic acetabulum may leave part of the component unsupported by native bone. Lack of support increases the stress at the bone-implant (or bone-cement) interface and thus may increase the probability of mechanical failure. The native bone has to support at least 70% of the surface area of component to give stability and allow adequate ingrowth on bone.[10] When sufficient coverage of the implant by native bone cannot be achieved with standard acetabular implant placement, an alternative reconstructive technique should be considered.

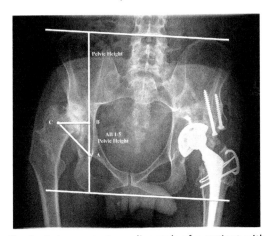

Fig. 1. Anteroposterior radiograph of a patient with DDH depicting the references lines and true acetabular region based on the method by Ranawat and colleagues.[8]

Cemented Acetabular Components with and Without Augmentation

High incidence of mechanical failure rates has been reported for cemented acetabular components implanted without structural augmentation (ie, supported by cement only), intentional elevation or medialization at long term. Reported failure rates have varied from 16% to 52% at a mean follow-up of approximately 10 to 20 years.[5,9,11,12] Younger age at surgery, severe hip dysplasia with extensive proximal migration of the femoral head, and nonanatomic placement of the acetabular component correlated with a poor outcome in these studies. Others have reported low wear, revision, and loosening rates resulting from the use of cemented Charnley offset-bore components.[13]

The literature demonstrates that when cemented acetabular components are used and cup coverage is required, the cup should not be augmented with cement. Autogenous bone graft augmentation in association with cemented acetabular components for hip dysplasia has provided satisfactory early clinical results, but a higher rate of failure with longer follow-up and with increasing revision rates due to graft collapse, particularly when a large amount of the socket is supported by graft, or due to socket loosening is observed.[10,14–19] At 10 to 11 years, about 40% of cemented acetabular components partly supported by autograft show radiographic signs of loosening, and 10% to 20% have been revised.[10,19] Similarly, Lee and colleagues[17] noted an increase in the graft failure rate of 36 cemented cups from 6% at 5 years to 39% at 10 years. Better results have been reported when the hip center initially is restored to its anatomic position,[20] when the graft supports less than 30% to 40% of the component, and when posterior as well as superior support is provided.[10,19] More recently, Kobayashi and colleagues[21] noted excellent clinical results with no hip radiographic evidence of failure of fixation at 19 years with a cemented cup. Large bone grafts in association with cemented sockets have not provided optimal long-term durability; however, when the reconstruction fails, the bone graft usually provides additional bone stock restoration and facilitates subsequent revision surgery. The use of cemented acetabular components along with impacted femoral head autograft contained with mesh is a viable option and has shown a cumulative survival of the cup with revision for any reason as the end point of 96% at 10 years and 84% at 15 years.[22] The technique of cup cementation, however, requires experience and precision and in North America has fallen out of favor. One cannot ignore, however, that the major advantage of using cemented all polyethylene components in the young patient population is related to relatively low polyethylene wear rates.

Cementless Acetabular Components Without Augmentation

There are several techniques that can be used if a cementless ingrowth acetabular component is preferred. Cementless designs have shown long lasting ingrowth potential. Anderson and Harris[23] reported on 20 dysplastic hips reconstructed with an uncemented hemispheric cup and followed for a mean of 6.9 years. Native bone covered 75% to 100% of the components that were placed an average of 28 mm (range, 5–66 mm) proximal to the interteardrop line (ie, some of these were high hip centers). None of the sockets had been revised and none had loosening, migration, osteolysis, or complete radiolucent lines, demonstrating that uncemented reconstruction is a viable option in the dysplastic hip. Longer follow-up of a greater number of patients is required before uncemented sockets can definitively be said to outperform cemented cups in dysplastic hips because polyethylene wear has shown to limit the success of cementless reconstruction. Slight elevation of hip center to achieve coverage is an acceptable form of reconstruction in select cases (**Fig. 2**).

High Hip Center

Several techniques to manage severe bone deficiency problems have been described including superior placement of the cup.[9,24,25] Intentional proximal placement of the acetabular component was recommended by Russotti and Harris[25] for patients in whom the placement of the acetabular component in the true anatomic position would otherwise require grafts to provide most of the socket's structural support. The investigators reported revision and loosening rates of 2.7% and 16%, respectively, in a group of complex cemented

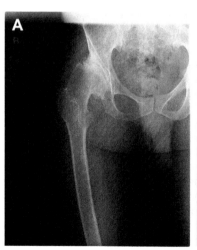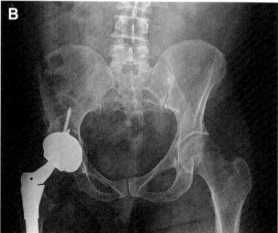

Fig. 2. (A) Preoperative radiograph of a 44-year-old man with long standing right hip dysplasia with subluxation. Reconstruction was performed with a cementless cup obtaining good coverage without head autograft. (B) Postoperative radiograph of a 44-year-old man with long standing right hip dysplasia with subluxation. Reconstruction was performed with a cementless cup obtaining good coverage without head autograft.

total hip replacements that included 19 dysplastic hips. Schutzer and Harris[26] later reported the results of superiorly placed uncemented components in a mixed group of 56 hips that included only 5 primary arthroplasties on dysplastic hips. At a mean follow-up of 3.3 years, no acetabular component had been revised for loosening. These 2 studies suggest that proximal placement of both cemented and uncemented acetabular components did not negatively affect the outcome of acetabular reconstruction provided that the component was not lateralized. However, other reports support the placement of acetabular components in the true acetabular region. Higher loosening and revision rates for both femoral and acetabular components have been reported in several series when cemented acetabular cups are initially placed superior or lateral to the anatomic position.[9,20] Proximal placement of the acetabular component probably should be reserved for the elderly patient in whom an anatomic position would leave more than 40% to 50% of the socket surface uncovered or covered by bone graft.

Acetabular Component Medialization

Intentional medialization of the acetabular component through the medial wall by reaming or creating a controlled comminuted fracture has been reported to provide reasonable midterm results.[7,27] Low revision rates have been published combining this technique with both cemented[7] and uncemented[27] components followed up for an average of 7 years. However, nonprogressive but complete radiolucent lines greater than 1-mm wide were found around 18% of the cemented acetabular cups.[7] In reviewing their results with press-fit uncemented acetabular components inserted after reaming the medial acetabular wall, Dorr and colleagues[27] recommend creating a medial wall defect of about 25% of the acetabular area. Of 24 hips followed up for a mean of 7 years, 2 required polyethylene exchange, but none of the metal shells were revised or found radiographically to be loose. The average medialization of the hip center was 12.7 mm, and supplemental structural bone graft covering 15% to 30% of the component was used in only 6 hips. Long-term follow-up of the durability of this form of reconstruction in conjunction with uncemented cups is needed to demonstrate whether its advantages (technical simplicity and good lateral support of the cup on native bone) outweigh the undesirable loss of remaining medial acetabular bone stock. The authors do not recommend overmedialization of the acetabular component at the time of THA in patients with hip dysplasia. Slight medialization of the acetabulum may prevent the use of femoral head autograft in select cases (**Fig. 3**).

Acetabular Medial Wall Osteotomy

This technique, developed to medialize the acetabular component toward the optimal center of rotation and to maximize bony coverage, allows the usage of largest acetabular component possible to achieve good stability and minimize polyethylene wear. The method preserves medial wall trabecular bone stock and maintains the uniformity of the entire bone floor.[28] The authors think these important characteristics will help simplify future revision surgery, if required. One contraindication for the technique is an acetabular medial wall thickness of less than 10 mm. If the

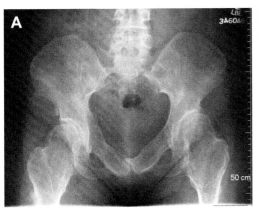
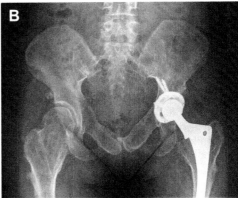

Fig. 3. (A) Preoperative radiograph of a 32-year-old with osteochondromatosis. Reconstruction was performed with medialization for coverage without the use of graft. (B) Postoperative radiograph of a 32-year-old with osteochondromatosis. Reconstruction was performed with medialization for coverage without the use of graft.

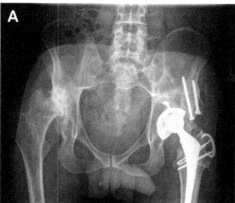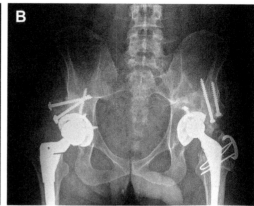

Fig. 4. (*A*) Preoperative radiograph of a 42-year-old man with left THA 20 years previously, no pain and some polyethylene wear. Right side was painful, low dislocation type acetabulum requiring reconstruction with femoral head autograft. (*B*) Postoperative radiograph of a 42-year-old man with left THA 20 years previously, no pain and some polyethylene wear. Right side was painful, low dislocation type acetabulum requiring reconstruction with femoral head autograft.

bony floor is thinner than 10 mm, it is difficult to perform the cork-shaped osteotomy and the bony fragment tends to be unstable. Zhang and colleagues[28] reported on 26 patients (30 hips) who were followed for mean period of 22 months. They reported restoration of hip biomechanical environment and suggested this technique as a reliable form of obtaining acetabular coverage in the dysplastic hip.

Cementless Acetabular Components with Augmentation

Literature on the usage of lateral bone graft augmentation in association with uncemented acetabular components have shown excellent results with 85% of the acetabular components free of revision for any cause at 10 years with minimal resorption of the bone autograft.[29] Furthermore, the use of autogenous bone grafts and cementless cups have been shown to successfully restore the patient's own bone and substantially augment the pelvic bone stock in the majority of patients at 8 to 15 years.[30] Unpublished data from the Mayo Clinic have showed 68% of survival of the acetabular component from acetabular revision due to aseptic loosening at 20 years. At the time of revision surgery, all autogenous femoral heads had united with reconstitution of the previous anterolateral bone deficiency (**Figs. 4**A and **4**B).

The authors' preferred treatment:

1. Restore center of rotation as close as possible to the native hip center.
2. Uncemented acetabular fixation. The anteroposterior dimension of the native acetabulum dictates the size of the acetabular component.
3. In subluxation, slight medialization of hip center of rotation usually avoids the use of bulk autograft for reconstruction.
4. In low hip dislocation, socket uncoverage will usually require augmentation of femoral head autograft.
5. In high dislocation, a small uncemented acetabular component without autograft coverage is often the best option because complete coverage is usually obtained within the anterior and posterior walls of the native bony acetabulum.
6. Because of their wear characteristics, alternative bearing surfaces, such as highly crosslinked polyethylene and ceramic, are often used in younger patients.

REFERENCES

1. Guille JT, Pizzutillo PD, MacEwen GD. Development dysplasia of the hip from birth to six months. J Am Acad Orthop Surg 2000;8(4):232–42.
2. Cooperman DR, Wallensten R, Stulberg SD. Acetabular dysplasia in the adult. Clin Orthop Relat Res 1983;(175):79–85.
3. Harris WH. Etiology of osteoarthritis of the hip. Clin Orthop Relat Res 1986;(213):20–33.
4. Weinstein SL, Mubarak SJ, Wenger DR. Developmental hip dysplasia and dislocation: part I. Instr Course Lect 2004;53:523–30.
5. Sochart DH, Porter ML. The long-term results of Charnley low-friction arthroplasty in young patients who have congenital dislocation, degenerative osteoarthrosis, or rheumatoid arthritis. J Bone Joint Surg Am 1997;79(11):1599–617.

6. Crowe JF, Mani VJ, Ranawat CS. Total hip replacement in congenital dislocation and dysplasia of the hip. J Bone Joint Surg Am 1979;61(1):15–23.

7. Hartofilakidis G, Satmos K, Karachalios T, et al. Congenital hip disease in adults. Classification of acetabular deficiencies and operative treatment with acetabuloplasty combined with total hip arthroplasty. J Bone Joint Surg Am 1996;78(5):683–92.

8. Ranawat CS, Dorr LD, Inglis AE. Total hip arthroplasty in protrusio acetabuli of rheumatoid arthritis. J Bone Joint Surg Am 1980;62(7):1059–65.

9. Pagnano W, Hanssen AD, Lewallen DG, et al. The effect of superior placement of the acetabular component on the rate of loosening after total hip arthroplasty. J Bone Joint Surg Am 1996;78(7):1004–14.

10. Mulroy RD Jr, Harris WH. Failure of acetabular autogenous grafts in total hip arthroplasty. Increasing incidence: a follow-up note. J Bone Joint Surg Am 1990;72(10):1536–40.

11. MacKenzie JR, Kelley SS, Johnston RC. Total hip replacement for coxarthrosis secondary to congenital dysplasia and dislocation of the hip. Long-term results. J Bone Joint Surg Am 1996;78(1):55–61.

12. Numair J, Joshi AB, Murphy JC, et al. Total hip arthroplasty for congenital dysplasia or dislocation of the hip. Survivorship analysis and long-term results. J Bone Joint Surg Am 1997;79(9):1352–60.

13. Ioannidis TT, Zacharakis N, Magnissalis EA, et al. Long-term behaviour of the Charnley offset-bore acetabular cup. J Bone Joint Surg Br 1998;80(1):48–53.

14. Gerber SD, Harris WH. Femoral head autografting to augment acetabular deficiency in patients requiring total hip replacement. A minimum five-year and an average seven-year follow-up study. J Bone Joint Surg Am 1986;68(8):1241–8.

15. Gross AE, Catre MG. The use of femoral head autograft shelf reconstruction and cemented acetabular components in the dysplastic hip. Clin Orthop Relat Res 1994;(298):60–6.

16. Inao S, Matsuno T. Cemented total hip arthroplasty with autogenous acetabular bone grafting for hips with developmental dysplasia in adults: the results at a minimum of ten years. J Bone Joint Surg Br 2000;82(3):375–7.

17. Lee BP, Cabanela ME, Wallrichs SL, et al. Bone-graft augmentation for acetabular deficiencies in total hip arthroplasty. Results of long-term follow-up evaluation. J Arthroplasty 1997;12(5):503–10.

18. Ritter MA, Trancik TM. Lateral acetabular bone graft in total hip arthroplasty. A three- to eight-year follow-up study without internal fixation. Clin Orthop Relat Res 1985;(193):156–9.

19. Rodriguez JA, Huk OL, Pellicci PM, et al. Autogenous bone grafts from the femoral head for the treatment of acetabular deficiency in primary total hip arthroplasty with cement. Long-term results. J Bone Joint Surg Am 1995;77(8):1227–33.

20. Stans AA, Pagnano MW, Shaughnessy WJ, et al. Results of total hip arthroplasty for Crowe Type III developmental hip dysplasia. Clin Orthop Relat Res 1998;(348):149–57.

21. Kobayashi S, Saito N, Nawata M, et al. Total hip arthroplasty with bulk femoral head autograft for acetabular reconstruction in developmental dysplasia of the hip. J Bone Joint Surg Am 2003; 85(4):615–21.

22. Somford MP, Bolder SB, Gardeniers JW, et al. Favorable survival of acetabular reconstruction with bone impaction grafting in dysplastic hips. Clin Orthop Relat Res 2008;466(2):359–65.

23. Anderson MJ, Harris WH. Total hip arthroplasty with insertion of the acetabular component without cement in hips with total congenital dislocation or marked congenital dysplasia. J Bone Joint Surg Am 1999;81(3):347–54.

24. McQueary FG, Johnston RC. Coxarthrosis after congenital dysplasia. Treatment by total hip arthroplasty without acetabular bone-grafting. J Bone Joint Surg Am 1988;70(8):1140–4.

25. Russotti GM, Harris WH. Proximal placement of the acetabular component in total hip arthroplasty. A long-term follow-up study. J Bone Joint Surg Am 1991;73(4):587–92.

26. Schutzer SF, Harris WH. High placement of porous-coated acetabular components in complex total hip arthroplasty. J Arthroplasty 1994;9(4):359–67.

27. Dorr LD, Tawakkol S, Moorthy M, et al. Medial protrusio technique for placement of a porous-coated, hemispherical acetabular component without cement in a total hip arthroplasty in patients who have acetabular dysplasia. J Bone Joint Surg Am 1999;81(1):83–92.

28. Zhang H, Huang Y, Zhou YX, et al. Acetabular medial wall displacement osteotomy in total hip arthroplasty: a technique to optimize the acetabular reconstruction in acetabular dysplasia. J Arthroplasty 2005;20(5): 562–7.

29. Spangehl MJ, Berry DJ, Trousdale RT, et al. Uncemented acetabular components with bulk femoral head autograft for acetabular reconstruction in developmental dysplasia of the hip: results at five to twelve years. J Bone Joint Surg Am 2001; 83(10):1484–9.

30. Farrell CM, Berry DJ, Cabanela ME. Autogenous femoral head bone grafts for acetabular deficiency in total-hip arthroplasty for developmental dysplasia of the hip: long-term effect on pelvic bone stock. J Arthroplasty 2005;20(6):698–702.

Femoral Considerations for Total Hip Replacement in Hip Dysplasia

Kevin I. Perry, MD, Daniel J. Berry, MD*

KEYWORDS

• Hypoplasia • Femur • Deformity

KEY POINTS

- The common deformities in the dysplastic femur include hypoplasia, excessive neck anteversion, a valgus neck-shaft angle, metaphyseal-diaphyseal mismatch, and a posteriorly displaced greater trochanter.
- Depending on the degree of hip dysplasia, where the cup is placed, and length of the opposite leg, management of leg length on the femoral side is also a frequent challenge.
- Although often thought of as an acetabular deformity, hip dysplasia also usually has associated femoral bone deformity.

INTRODUCTION

Developmental dysplasia of the hip (DDH) is one of the most common conditions leading to secondary arthritis of the hip (**Fig. 1**).[1,2] After nonarthroplasty options are exhausted, many patients with symptomatic arthritis secondary to dysplasia become candidates for total hip replacement. There is a predictable spectrum of femoral and acetabular abnormalities that must be considered when contemplating total hip arthroplasty (THA) in the patient with DDH. This article presents the specific considerations related to femoral reconstruction during THA in patients with hip dysplasia.

Milder cases of bone deformity present little difference from standard approaches to femoral reconstruction. In contrast, more severe bone and soft tissue deformities can present a multitude of issues including hypoplasia of the femur, excessive femoral anteversion, a valgus neck-shaft angle, metaphyseal-diaphyseal mismatch, a posteriorly displaced greater trochanter, and challenges related to leg length.

Preoperative radiographs with magnification markers should be obtained on all dysplastic patients who are being considered for THA. The surgeon should look carefully at these films to assess for signs associated with the dysplastic femur. Specific elements to scrutinize are the amount of proximal migration of the femoral head, the location of the greater trochanter, the size of the femoral canal, and overall femoral morphology. It is difficult to assess the amount of femoral anteversion without the use of three-dimensional imaging, although marked abnormalities frequently are identifiable on plain films. Although it is not the routine practice of the authors, three-dimensional imaging may be obtained if understanding the amount of anteversion before surgery will assist the surgeon.

DDH may be classified according to several systems. The most common is that of Crowe and colleagues[3] based on the extent of radiographic proximal migration of the femoral head. The extent of subluxation does correlate with the degree of femoral deformity, but not predictably. Robertson and colleagues[4] were the first to use computed tomography (CT) scans to study the morphology of the dysplastic femur. They evaluated 24 hips with DDH and found that femoral anteversion

Department of Orthopedic Surgery, Mayo Clinic, 200 First Street Southwest, Rochester, MN 55905, USA
* Corresponding author.
E-mail address: berry.daniel@mayo.edu

Orthop Clin N Am 43 (2012) 377–386
doi:10.1016/j.ocl.2012.05.010
0030-5898/12/$ – see front matter © 2012 Published by Elsevier Inc.

orthopedic.theclinics.com

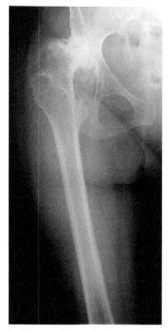

Fig. 1. Typical femoral morphology of DDH.

control group, the dysplastic femurs had shorter necks, smaller intramedullary canals, and 10° to 14° more anteversion independent of the amount of subluxation of the hip. Noble and colleagues[8] reported on 154 women with DDH and found that patients with more advanced subluxation (Crowe III and IV) had increased hypoplasia of the femur, deformity of the femoral head, and straighter femoral canals with thinner cortices. However, even those femurs with mild subluxation (Crowe I) had measurable alterations in the anatomy of their proximal femur. Argenson and colleagues[9] reviewed the radiographs and CT scans of 83 hips with DDH and compared femoral morphology with a control group. The intramedullary femoral canal had reduced dimensions in the mediolateral and anteroposterior planes in all patients with DDH compared with the control group. There was no correlation between femoral morphology and Crowe class.

TECHNICAL CHALLENGES UNIQUE TO FEMORAL RECONSTRUCTION IN DDH

The anatomic abnormalities of the dysplastic femur are numerous and present reconstructive challenges to the surgeon. In addition, patients frequently have undergone previous nonarthroplasty procedures that have altered their already distorted anatomy. It is important to be familiar with the patient's previous procedures, because sometimes canal realignment procedures must take place concomitantly with THA (**Fig. 2**). For example, valgus subtrochanteric (Schantz) osteotomy, can present considerable difficulty in femoral reconstruction during THA.

extended down through the metaphysis to the level of the lesser trochanter. In accordance with previous studies,[5,6] in the diaphysis, the femoral canal was wider in the anterior to posterior direction than in the medial to lateral direction. The extent of femoral deformity was not significantly influenced by the extent of disease as classified by Crowe and colleagues.[3] Sugano and colleagues[7] also used three-dimensional CT reconstructions to study the morphology of 35 dysplastic hips compared with a matched cohort. Compared with the

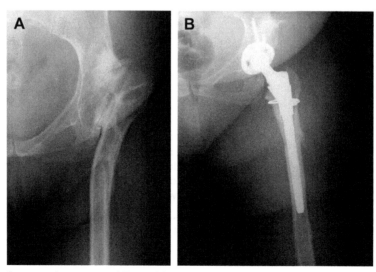

Fig. 2. Deformity from previous surgery (A) requiring corrective osteotomy (B).

Exposure

Several operative approaches can be performed safely for THA in patients with hip dysplasia. For mild dysplasia, adequate exposure usually can be obtained through any of the popular approaches to the hip including direct anterior, anterolateral, or the posterior approach, based on surgeon preference. Subtrochanteric osteotomy may be used to adjust femoral anteversion or to shorten the femur. This osteotomy also provides exposure of the acetabulum in cases of high hip dislocation. Greater trochanteric osteotomy or a trochanteric slide may be used in selected situations in which the hip cannot be dislocated or exposed with a traditional soft tissue exposure or in which greater trochanteric repositioning is desirable to restore hip biomechanics.

Restoration of abductor function is crucial to the success of THA in the dysplastic hip. The proximal displacement of the femoral head relative to the true acetabulum and excessive femoral neck anteversion can cause severe distortion of the length and direction of the abductor muscle fibers.[10] This distortion must be considered during the operative approach to avoid proceeding through improper planes of dissection. The abductors are often underdeveloped and more transverse in nature than normal. This distortion of the abductor muscles can severely affect their function, making them less efficient. Restoration of the hip to its true hip center and correction of femoral neck anteversion can often provide more normal abductor anatomy and function. Specific techniques to restore length and position of the greater trochanter are discussed later.

Canal Diameter and Shape

Charnley and Feagin[2] showed that the canal of the dysplastic femur is often extremely narrow and is frequently an exaggerated oval in cross section, wider anterior to posterior than medial to lateral. This shape complicates canal preparation. It is imperative to measure the size of the intramedullary canal before surgery to ensure that appropriately sized and shaped femoral components are available at the time of surgery. Proper component sizing minimizes the risk of fracture (or perforation) during canal preparation and seating of the femoral component.

Anteversion

Femoral neck anteversion is defined as the angle between the transverse axis of the knee and the transverse axis of the femoral neck.[11] Femoral anteversion varies widely in patients with DDH.[12] Three-dimensional imaging is a reliable method to accurately assess the amount of femoral neck anteversion, which can reach as much as 90°. Surgeons must be prepared to deal with a varying degree of anteversion encountered at the time of surgery. If excessive femoral anteversion in the dysplastic femur is not recognized, excessive anteversion of the femoral component may ensue and can lead to intraprosthetic impingement, (anterior) hip instability, or an internal rotation gait that is not well tolerated by patients.

Minor or moderate degrees of femoral anteversion abnormality can be corrected during THA using certain standard implants and methods of fixation. In cases of more severe anteversion abnormalities, there are 2 effective methods of correction: subtrochanteric osteotomy; and special, uncemented stems (either modular or conical with flutes). With a subtrochanteric osteotomy, the goal is to rotate the proximal fragment such that the metaphyseal flare and the greater trochanter are placed into a more anatomic position. This position helps restore anatomic and functional characteristics of the abductors and also minimizes the risk of impingement of the trochanter on the pelvis. Furthermore, this repositions the metaphyseal flare to a position that accommodates the triangular metaphyseal portion of a femoral component.

Leg Length

In many patients with DDH, it is desirable and/or necessary to lengthen the operative extremity by placing the acetabular component in an anatomic location, particularly in unilateral cases with a short leg or bilateral cases with higher levels of subluxation/dislocation. One concern associated with lengthening that has been shown repeatedly[13–16] is risk of palsies of the sciatic or femoral nerves.

Dunn and Hess[10] suggested that it was safe to lengthen the limb by 5 to 7 cm in the setting of dysplasia. In their series, 13 of 22 hips were lengthened by at least 5 cm (range 5–9.2 cm). None of the patients in this series with limbs lengthened by more than 5 cm experienced a nerve palsy. The 1 patient who developed a (sciatic) nerve palsy was lengthened by 4 cm.

In a report by Edwards and colleagues,[17] 23 hips out of 614 consecutive THAs experienced either a peroneal or sciatic nerve palsy. Twenty-two percent of these patients had an underlying diagnosis of DDH. This study was the first to show a relationship between the amount of lengthening and the development of a nerve palsy. Peroneal nerve palsies were associated with limb lengthening of 3.8 cm or less, and sciatic nerve palsies were associated with lengthening of 4.0 cm or more. These data have yet to be corroborated.

In their review of 3126 consecutive THAs, Schmalzried and colleagues[13] found a 5.2% incidence of nerve palsies in patients with DDH. Of the 9 patients with DDH who experienced a nerve palsy, 6 had their limbs lengthened by more than 3.0 cm. Of all 52 patients who experienced a nerve palsy in this study, 13 patients had their operative extremity lengthened by more than 2.5 cm. The investigators concluded that limb lengthening is a major contributor to nerve palsy after THA, but failed to identify the specific parameters of lengthening that should be avoided.

Farrell and colleagues[18] reported on 27,004 consecutive primary THAs performed at Mayo Clinic (not all for DDH) and found that, in 43 patients with a (sciatic, peroneal, or femoral) nerve injury, overall length of the extremity was increased by an average of 1.7 cm. A matched cohort without nerve injury had the operative limb lengthened by only 1.1 cm. A conditional, logistical regression analysis showed that patients with increased limb lengthening were at increased risk for nerve injury.

Although the amount of lengthening that causes nerve dysfunction is not known, if templating suggests that reducing the femur into an anatomically placed acetabular component lengthens the limb by more than 3 to 4 cm, the authors typically consider shortening of the femur to reduce the amount of leg lengthening. Intraoperative electromyographic monitoring may also be considered in these cases, although its value in reducing risk of nerve palsy is unproven.

RECONSTRUCTION OPTIONS: CROWE TYPE I TO III DDH
Cemented Stems

Cemented femoral components are appealing because they are versatile and allow the surgeon to address many of the anteversion and deformity issues encountered in DDH. The advantages of cemented stems are that (1) they do not rely on an exact fit in the metaphysis or diaphysis, (2) they can be cemented in varying degrees of version (compensating for mild or moderate version abnormalities), and (3) cemented implants are typically smaller than uncemented implants and are therefore easier to fit into the smaller diaphyses of dysplastic femurs. The drawbacks of the cemented technique are that (1) dysplastic patients are often younger and many North American surgeons prefer uncemented implants in young patients,[19] and (2) dysplastic femora with severe version abnormalities cannot be fully corrected with cemented components without rotational osteotomy.

Selected cemented stems have shown excellent midterm success[2] in hip dysplasia. In their review

of 232 dysplastic hips treated with cemented hip replacements, Numair and colleagues[20] showed a survivorship of 97% of the cemented femoral component at an average follow-up of 9.9 years. Anwar and colleagues[21] found similar midterm results in their review of 34 cemented total hip replacements in patients with DDH. At an average follow-up of 9.4 years, radiographic loosening was evident in only 3/34 (9%) femoral components. The investigators attributed these failures to poor cementing technique. In their review of 60 cemented THAs performed in 44 patients for hip dysplasia, Sochart and Porter[22] found that only 6 femoral components had been revised (for loosening) at an average of 20.3 years. Survival rates of the femoral component at 10 and 20 years were 97% and 89%, respectively.

Poorer results also have been reported.[23–25] In their review of 70 THAs done for Crowe type III dysplasia, Stans and colleagues[19] showed a 40% aseptic loosening rate of cemented femoral components at an average of 16 years' follow-up.

If cemented components are used, it is important to maintain a continuous cement mantle and to place the component in good overall alignment. To optimize the bone/cement interface, careful canal preparation is paramount. The femoral canal is prepared sequentially with broaches of increasing size. The broaches should be larger than the femoral component to allow for a proper cement mantle. After the final broaching has been performed, appropriate trials are placed in the canal and proper length and stability are confirmed. It is important to memorize the version of the trial component that provides maximum stability without impinging on the acetabulum so that this position can be easily repeated during femoral component insertion. A cement restrictor is then placed distally, ensuring enough room for a cement mantle distal to the femoral component. The femoral canal is then irrigated thoroughly using a pressurized lavage system, to improve interdigitation of the cement into the host bone. The canal is then dried in preparation for cementation. The investigators prefer to use epinephrine-soaked sponges to decrease bleeding from the host bone. After the cement has been prepared on the back table, it is inserted into a cement gun and injected into the femoral canal (distal to proximal). Once the canal has been filled with cement it should be pressurized to maximize interdigitation into the host bone. The stem is then carefully and slowly inserted, ensuring proper version of the component at all times. The cement is allowed to harden and then final modular head trialing is performed to optimize stability and length.

Proximally Coated Monoblock Stems

Many surgeons, particularly in North America, prefer uncemented femoral component fixation in the younger, more active DDH population. Proximally coated, monoblock stems may be used success-fully in some cases of mild deformity. The advantage of these stems is that fixation is achieved proximally in the femur and has the potential to preserve bone stock in the younger DDH population. Proximally coated stems rely on a congruent fit of the pros-thesis in the proximal femoral metaphysis. In cases of more severe femoral deformity (particularly a femur with a valgus or overly anteverted neck), these stems are difficult to insert without malsizing or creating implant malposition or bone fracture. To our knowledge, there are few published studies of the results of the proximally coated monoblock stem in the specific setting of hip dysplasia. Faldini and colleagues[26] recently reported on 28 patients (younger than 50 years) with DDH treated with a ce-mentless, tapered stem. At an average follow-up of 12 years, all patients had clinical improvements in functional outcomes and there was no evidence of loosening of any of the femoral components. The investigators concluded that the tapered stem is a suitable option for dysplastic patients despite their age at the time of THA.

The surgical technique for proximally coated stems differs from fully coated implants. Inherent to the success of these implants is intimate appo-sition of the implant-bone interface in the metaphy-sis of the femur. In the dysplastic femur, these stems can prove to be technically challenging because the metaphysis of the femur can have severe version abnormalities. Mating proximally coated stems with the metaphysis of the dysplastic femur frequently leads to excessive anteversion. These stems are indicated in only the mildly deformed femur.

Fully Coated Stems/Fluted Tapered Stems

Fully coated, monoblock, uncemented stems and fluted, tapered stems allow some adjustment of femoral anteversion because fixation is achieved distally and there is less reliance on a tight fit in the anteverted proximal femur. However, many sur-geons prefer to avoid using distally fixed stems in this younger patient population in hopes of pre-serving precious femoral bone stock for the future.

Wangen and colleagues[27] reviewed 28 patients with DDH (all less than 30 years of age) in whom an uncemented, straight stem fully coated with hydroxyapatite (HA) was used for femoral recon-struction. At an average of 13 years' follow-up, none of the femoral components had been revised and none had evidence of radiographic loosening.

They concluded that fully coated HA stems provide an excellent option for femoral reconstruc-tion in patients with DDH.

The goal of femoral preparation in the setting of fully coated porous implants is to intimately mate the femoral component with the prepared femur. The canal should be prepared first with sequential reaming. The starting point in the proximal femur is critical to prevent reaming in varus/valgus or flexion/extension. Most systems encourage slight under-reaming of the femoral canal (relative to the implant) to provide a scratch fit of the diaphy-seal portion of the femoral component. Often, in the dysplastic femur, the scratch fit can only be achieved in the medial to lateral direction because of the ovoid nature of the canal. The metaphysis is then broached to the size of the desired compo-nent, ensuring proper version of the component throughout the broaching process. It is important to recognize the degree of anteversion abnor-mality of the host femur because fully coated stems allow only modest correction of version abnormalities. After the femur has been properly reamed and broached, a trial femoral component may be used to check limb lengths and stability before the final femoral component is inserted.

Modular Stems

In many cases in which there is more than mild deformity, many North American surgeons have moved toward using modular, uncemented stems; these allow unlimited adjustment of version and address the metaphyseal-diaphyseal mismatch frequently encountered in DDH (**Fig. 3**). Modularity of the stem allows the surgeon to independently match the anatomy of the metaphyseal and diaph-yseal bone with the hope that more intimate contact between the host bone and the prosthesis will lead to better long-term outcomes. The main drawbacks of modularity concern the strength of the modular junctions[28,29] and fretting or corrosion of these junctions.

In their review of 175 dysplastic hips, Christie and colleagues[30] found that a modular femoral compo-nent with a separate proximal sleeve and body had excellent midterm results, with 98% showing stable bone ingrowth radiographically at an average of 5.3 years. In their series of 28 Crowe type III and IV dysplastic hips, Biant and colleagues[31] showed excellent 10-year results with the use of a modular stem. All patients showed improved functional outcomes and, at the time of last follow-up, none of the 28 stems had been revised.

Successful implantation of modular stems is favored by an intimate fit of the metaphyseal sleeve and secure press fit of the stem distally.

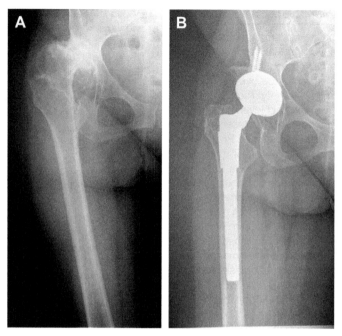

Fig. 3. Modular THA.

Femoral preparation begins with distal reaming of the femur. Sequential reaming is performed until firm cortical contact is achieved across several centimeters of the femoral canal. It is important to recognize that, because of the oval shape of the femur in the dysplastic femur, it is common to achieve cortical contact with the medial and lateral cortices before the anterior and posterior cortices. Excessive reaming of the medial and lateral cortices in an attempt to make cortical contact with the anterior and posterior cortices should be avoided. Attention is turned next to the proximal femur. Proximal reaming with conical reamers should be performed until contact has been made with cortical bone, which usually occurs first in the anterior femoral cortex. Next, the metaphyseal flare is milled with system-specific instrumentation, again until cortical contact has been achieved. Trial components can then be inserted to optimize version, length, and offset. The final proximal sleeve is inserted first and should be seated so that rotational and axial stability are achieved in the metaphysis. The stem is then inserted, ensuring proper version before the taper is engaged.

Modular stems may be considered in dysplastic patients with moderate to severe rotational deformity of the proximal femur because the proximal sleeve can be inserted in any version without affecting the final version of the stem. These stems also may be used in the setting of femoral osteotomy because they provide excellent angular and rotational stability both proximal and distal to a subtrochanteric osteotomy.

Custom Implants

Deformity of the proximal femur and a small intramedullary canal occasionally precludes the use of an off-the-shelf femoral component and calls for a custom implant. The advantage of a custom femoral component is that the deformity of the femur can be specifically addressed with an implant that is designed for the particular femur being reconstructed. A component that ideally optimizes bone-prosthesis contact (if uncemented) and abductor mechanics, and corrects for version abnormalities, is designed. Drawbacks of custom prostheses include cost, time to production, and limited options available at the time of surgery.

In their review of 19 dysplastic hips treated with cemented, custom implants by Huo and colleagues,[32] patients had excellent clinical results at an average follow-up of 57 months. No stem in this series had been revised at the time of last follow-up, although 2 stems did show radiographic signs consistent with loosening.

Sakai and colleagues[33] also showed favorable results with the use of a custom stem in dysplastic hips. In their review of 99 dysplastic hips in which a custom implant was used, only 1 femoral component had been revised (for aseptic loosening) at an average of 9.3 years.

RECONSTRUCTIVE OPTIONS: CROWE TYPE IV DDH

In more severe cases of DDH (Crowe type IV), femoral shortening may be necessary to avoid excessive stretch of the sciatic nerve (see **Fig. 1**). The authors typically lengthen the operative extremity only enough to provide good stability and function of the extremity. Shortening of the femur can be accomplished by 1 of 2 popular methods: sequential resection of the proximal femur or subtrochanteric shortening osteotomy.

Sequential Resection of the Proximal Femur

Sequential resection of the proximal femur allows small, incremental adjustments to limb length, which does not necessitate the same careful preoperative planning as the subtrochanteric shortening osteotomy. Nevertheless, it has several major disadvantages: first, it requires a greater trochanteric osteotomy that must be reattached to a tube of cortical bone. As a result, nonunion rates are high. Second, the tubular shape of the remaining femur after sequential resection precludes the use of most uncemented stems and leaves a new permanent femoral deformity.

In sequential resection of the proximal femur, a greater trochanteric osteotomy must be performed to preserve the hip abductors. After this has been accomplished, the proximal femur is sequentially resected until length is optimized. Frequent trialing of the femoral component between sequential resections ensures that enough femur is preserved to provide stability of the hip. A small, cemented DDH stem (with little metaphyseal flare) is usually used because the remaining femur is only a straight tube with little metaphysis to mate with the femoral component.

In their series of 22 high hip dislocations treated with sequential resection of the proximal femur, Dunn and Hess[10] had difficulty seating the final femoral component in 8 hips. They attributed this difficulty to the tight fit of the femoral component in the canal.

Subtrochanteric Osteotomy

Subtrochanteric osteotomy of the femur provides the opportunity to simultaneously address several of the issues encountered in THA for the dysplastic hip (**Figs. 4** and **5**). It allows derotation of excessive femoral anteversion (if present), which facilitates better position of the greater trochanter and can result in better abductor mechanics. Subtrochanteric osteotomy also preserves the proximal femoral metaphysis, allowing simpler insertion of certain uncemented femoral components. In addition, with an additional shortening osteotomy, subtrochanteric osteotomy also allows femoral shortening, which can correct limb length discrepancies and protect the sciatic nerve from excessive stretch.

In their series of 18 dysplastic hips treated with shortening, derotational subtrochanteric osteotomy with a cemented polished tapered

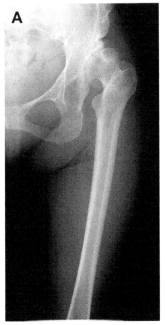 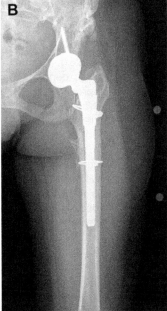

Fig. 4. Subtrochanteric shortening osteotomy.

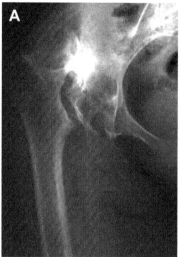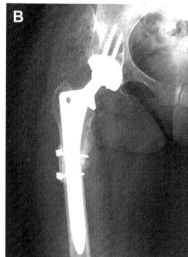

Fig. 5. Subtrochanteric shortening osteotomy.

stem, Charity and colleagues[34] showed excellent midterm outcomes. All patients showed improvement in overall pain scores, and, at an average follow-up of 114 months, only 1 hip had been revised (for osteotomy nonunion).

In the setting of reconstruction for high hip dislocation (Crowe IV), the authors prefer to use an uncemented femoral component in conjunction with a subtrochanteric shortening osteotomy, which is an elegant solution that also allows the surgeon to correct proximal femoral deformity if present (see **Fig. 2**). The subtrochanteric osteotomy is performed according to the technique described by Krych and colleagues.[35] In this technique, the femoral neck cut is made based on preoperative templating and the intramedullary canal of the proximal fragment is provisionally reamed and broached before the first osteotomy. Next, a transverse proximal femoral osteotomy is performed distal to the lesser trochanter, approximately 10 cm distal to the tip of the greater trochanter. This stage can be done before acetabular preparation to help with exposure, as described earlier. Once acetabular preparation is complete, a trial component is placed into the proximal femoral segment and the hip (consisting of only the trial stem in the proximal segment of bone) is reduced. The amount of femoral shortening needed can be estimated by the amount of overlap between the proximal and distal segments when gentle traction is applied to the limb and from preoperative planning. The second, more distal femoral osteotomy can then be performed based on this measurement and preoperative templating. Slightly less femur is usually resected than was planned so that additional resection may be performed to

adjust the limb length or provide better osteotomy apposition before the femoral component insertion. After the segment has been removed, the femoral component is inserted into the proximal segment and advanced into the distal segment, which reduces the 2 fragments. The intercalary segment that has been removed is then split and used as an onlay autograft held in place by cables (see **Fig. 5**).

Yasgur and colleagues[36] showed excellent clinical results in 9 dysplastic patients undergoing hip arthroplasty with concomitant subtrochanteric shortening osteotomy. Eight of 9 patients went on to radiographic union of their osteotomy at an average of 5 months and all patients (including an asymptomatic nonunion) had good clinical outcomes. In a series of 28 Crowe IV dysplastic hips by Krych and colleagues,[37] THA performed in conjunction with subtrochanteric shortening osteotomy provided excellent clinical outcomes and a high rate of osteotomy union and implant fixation. Nevertheless, in congruence with previous reports, there was a higher rate of complications than is associated with primary THA done for degenerative arthritis.

SUMMARY

THA in the dysplastic hip is a technically demanding procedure that requires careful preoperative planning. The common deformities associated with the dysplastic femur include hypoplasia, excessive neck anteversion, a valgus neck-shaft angle, metaphyseal-diaphyseal mismatch, and a posteriorly displaced greater trochanter. In selected cases, osteotomy of the femur may be performed to correct anteversion and/or avoid excessive leg lengthening and stretch of the sciatic nerve. All of these issues mandate careful preoperative planning. With the advent of modern surgical techniques and implants, the bone deformities in hip dysplasia can be successfully addressed and THA has proved to be a successful and durable operation.

REFERENCES

1. Sanchez-Sotelo J, Trousdale RT, Berry DJ, et al. Surgical treatment of developmental dysplasia of the hip in adults: I. Nonarthroplasty options. J Am Acad Orthop Surg 2002;10(5):321–33.

2. Charnley J, Feagin JA. Low-friction arthroplasty in congenital subluxation of the hip. Clin Orthop Relat Res 1973;91:98–113.

3. Crowe JF, Mani VJ, Ranawat CS. Total hip replacement in congenital dislocation and dysplasia of the hip. J Bone Joint Surg Am 1979;61(1):15–23.

4. Robertson DD, Essinger JR, Imura S, et al. Femoral deformity in adults with developmental hip dysplasia. Clin Orthop 1996;327:196–206.

5. Mendes DG. Total hip arthroplasty in congenital dislocated hips. Clin Orthop 1981;161:63–79.

6. Gorski JM. Modular noncemented total hip arthroplasty for congenital dislocation of the hip. Case report and design rationale. Clin Orthop 1988;228:110–6.

7. Sugano N, Noble PC, Kamaric E, et al. The morphology of the femur in developmental dysplasia of the hip. J Bone Joint Surg Br 1998;80(4):711–9.

8. Noble PC, Kamaric E, Sugano N, et al. Three-dimensional shape of the dysplastic femur: implications for THR. Clin Orthop 2003;417:27–40.

9. Argenson JN, Ryembault E, Flecher S, et al. Three-dimensional anatomy of the hip in osteoarthritis after developmental dysplasia. J Bone Joint Surg Br 2005;87(9):1192–6.

10. Dunn HK, Hess WE. Total hip reconstruction in chronically dislocated hips. J Bone Joint Surg Am 1976;58(6):838–45.

11. Tonnis D, Heinecke A. Acetabular and femoral anteversion: relationship with osteoarthritis of the hip. J Bone Joint Surg Am 1999;81(12):1747–70.

12. Flecher X, Parratte S, Aubaniac JM, et al. Three-dimensional custom-designed cementless femoral stem for osteoarthritis secondary to congenital dislocation of the hip. J Bone Joint Surg Br 2007;89(12):1586–91.

13. Schmalzried TP, Amstutz HC, Dorey FJ. Nerve palsy associated with total hip replacement. Risk factors and prognosis. J Bone Joint Surg Am 1991;73(7):1074–80.

14. Solheim LF, Hagen R. Femoral and sciatic neuropathies after total hip arthroplasty. Acta Orthop Scand 1980;51(3):531–4.

15. Weber ER, Daube JR, Coventry MB. Peripheral neuropathies associated with total hip arthroplasty. J Bone Joint Surg Am 1976;58(1):66–9.

16. Nercessian OA, Piccoluga F, Eftekhar NS. Postoperative sciatic and femoral nerve palsy with reference to leg lengthening and medialization/lateralization of the hip joint following total hip arthroplasty. Clin Orthop 1994;304:165–71.

17. Edwards BN, Tullos HS, Noble PC. Contributory factors and etiology of sciatic nerve palsy in total hip arthroplasty. Clin Orthop 1987;218:136–41.

18. Farrell CM, Springer BD, Haidukewych GJ, et al. Motor nerve palsy following primary total hip arthroplasty. J Bone Joint Surg Am 2005;87(12):2619–25.

19. Stans AA, Pagnano MW, Shaughnessy WJ, et al. Results of total hip arthroplasty for Crowe type III developmental hip dysplasia. Clin Orthop 1998;348:149–57.

20. Numair J, Joshi AB, Murphy JC, et al. Total hip arthroplasty for congenital dysplasia or dislocation of the hip. Survivorship analysis and long-term results. J Bone Joint Surg Am 1997;79(9):1352–60.

21. Anwar MM, Sugano N, Masuhara K, et al. Total hip arthroplasty in the neglected congenital dislocation of the hip. A five- to 14-year follow-up study. Clin Orthop 1993;295:127–34.

22. Sochart DH, Porter ML. The long-term results of Charnley low-friction arthroplasty in young patients who have congenital dislocation, degenerative osteoarthrosis, or rheumatoid arthritis. J Bone Joint Surg Am 1997;79(11):1599–617.

23. Collis DK. Long-term (twelve to eighteen-year) follow-up of cemented total hip replacements in patients who were less than fifty years old. A follow-up note. J Bone Joint Surg Am 1991;73(4):593–7.

24. Randhawa K, Hossain FS, Smith B, et al. A prospective study of hip revision surgery using the Exeter long-stem prosthesis: function, subsidence, and complications for 57 patients. J Orthop Traumatol 2009;10(4):159–65.

25. Sporer SM, Callaghan JJ, Olejniczak JP, et al. Hybrid total hip arthroplasty in patients under the age of fifty: a five- to ten-year follow-up. J Arthroplasty 1998;13(5):485–91.

26. Faldini C, Miscione MT, Chehrassan M, et al. Congenital hip dysplasia treated by total hip arthroplasty using cementless tapered stem in patients younger than 50 years old: results after 12-years follow-up. J Orthop Trauma 2011;12(4):213–8.

27. Wangen H, Lereim P, Holm I, et al. Hip arthroplasty in patients younger than 30 years: excellent ten to 16-year follow-up results with a HA-coated stem. Int Orthop 2008;32(2):203–8.

28. Viceconti M, Ruggeri O, Toni A, et al. Design-related fretting wear in modular neck hip prosthesis. J Biomed Mater Res 1996;30(2):181–6.

29. Viceconti M, Baleani M, Squarzoni S, et al. Fretting wear in a modular neck hip prosthesis. J Biomed Mater Res 1997;35(2):207–16.

30. Christie MJ, DeBoer DK, Trick LW, et al. Primary total hip arthroplasty with use of the modular S-ROM prosthesis. Four to seven-year clinical and radiographic results. J Bone Joint Surg Am 1999;81(12):1707–16.

31. Biant LC, Bruce WJ, Assini JB, et al. Primary total hip arthroplasty in severe developmental dysplasia of the hip. Ten-year results using a cementless modular stem. J Arthroplasty 2009;24(1):27–32.

32. Huo MH, Salvati EA, Lieberman JR, et al. Custom-designed femoral prostheses in total hip arthroplasty done with cement for severe dysplasia of the hip. J Bone Joint Surg Am 1993;75(10):1497–504.

33. Sakai T, Sugano N, Ohzono K, et al. The custom femoral component is an effective option for congenital hip dysplasia. Clin Orthop 2006;451:146–53.

34. Charity JA, Tsiridis E, Sheeraz A, et al. Treatment of Crowe IV high hip dysplasia with total hip replacement using the Exeter stem and shortening derotational subtrochanteric osteotomy. J Bone Joint Surg Br 2011;93(1):34–8.

35. Krych AJ, Howard JL, Trousdale RT, et al. Total hip arthroplasty with shortening subtrochanteric osteotomy in Crowe type-IV developmental dysplasia: surgical technique. J Bone Joint Surg Am 2010;92(Suppl 1 Pt 2):176–87.

36. Yasgur DJ, Stuchin SA, Adler EM, et al. Subtrochanteric femoral shortening osteotomy in total hip arthroplasty for high-riding developmental dislocation of the hip. J Arthroplasty 1997;12(8):880–8.

37. Krych AJ, Howard JL, Trousdale RT, et al. Total hip arthroplasty with shortening subtrochanteric osteotomy in Crowe type-IV developmental dysplasia. J Bone Joint Surg Am 2009;91(9):2213–21.

Technical Considerations in Total Hip Arthroplasty After Femoral and Periacetabular Osteotomies

Adam A. Sassoon, MD, Robert T. Trousdale, MD*

KEYWORDS

- Total hip arthroplasty • Periacetabular osteotomy • Femoral osteotomy • Avascular necrosis

KEY POINTS

- Be prepared for broken hardware.
- Removal of extensive hardware can be avoided with proper implant selection.
- A staged approach for hardware removal before total hip arthroplasty (THA) is sometimes prudent.
- Critically assess the position of the greater trochanter preoperatively, so that a required osteotomy can be appropriately planned.
- Assess the femoral version preoperatively so that modular stems may be used if required.
- Recognize and prepare for femoral deformity that often accompanies acetabuli that have previously undergone an osteotomy.
- Be mindful of a retroverted socket after a previous acetabular osteotomy and plan accordingly.
- Overmedialization of the acetabulum may warrant additional fixation at the time of arthroplasty.

INTRODUCTION

Hip preservation surgery is often used to relieve pain and correct osseous deformity that would otherwise predispose patients to early-onset arthritis. Osteotomies of the proximal femur and acetabulum are performed in this setting to negate or, more commonly, prolong a patient's need to undergo a THA. Osteotomies are usually performed to address deformities of a congenital or developmental etiology; however, they are also used to address traumatic deformities, either during an initial presentation or in the treatment of nonunions/malunions. Osteotomies are also occasionally performed in the setting of avascular necrosis (AVN) and some other less common indications.

Despite a well-performed osteotomy and regardless of the impetus for its performance, a subsequent THA is sometimes required for progression of coxarthrosis. Previously performed osteotomies warrant deliberation in preoperative planning and patient counseling before conversion to an arthroplasty. The purpose of this article is to outline key technical considerations in the performance of THA after common osteotomies of both the proximal femur and acetabulum. Attention is called to retained hardware and anatomic variation, both innate and incurred.

THA AFTER FEMORAL OSTEOTOMY
Technical Pearls

Overview
Femoral osteotomies have been performed for a variety of indications, including but not limited to, congenital/developmental dysplasia, AVN, treatment of femoral neck fractures, treatment of proximal femoral nonunions/malunions, and osteoarthritis. In

Disclosures: funding sources—Dr Sassoon, none; Dr Trousdale, none; conflict of interest—Dr Sassoon, none; Dr Trousdale, none related to this article.
Department of Orthopedic Surgery, Mayo Clinic, 200 First Street Southwest, Rochester, MN 55905, USA
* Corresponding author.
E-mail address: trousdale.robert@mayo.edu

Orthop Clin N Am 43 (2012) 387–393
doi:10.1016/j.ocl.2012.05.006
0030-5898/12/$ – see front matter © 2012 Elsevier Inc. All rights reserved.

orthopedic.theclinics.com

most instances, these osteotomies are performed through the intertrochanteric region of the proximal femur to produce a more varus or valgus hip alignment, although purely rotational osteotomies may also be performed to alter the weight-bearing portion of the femoral head. Irrespective of the indication for femoral osteotomy, key technical considerations for subsequent THA include incision selection, hardware removal, abductor condition, femoral version, and femoral offset.

Incision selection

Most incisions for a varus-producing or valgus-producing osteotomy are longitudinal and centered over the greater trochanter. In these cases, the incision for an anterolateral, direct lateral, or posterior approach to the hip usually incorporates and uses the previous incision. In a series of 215 THAs after failed trochanteric osteotomies, the ideal arthroplasty incision was compromised in fewer than 5% of cases.[1] A direct anterior approach may be performed based on surgeon preference; however, this generally requires a separate incision for hardware removal. These incisions should be appropriately spread to allow for a skin bridge of at least 6 cm. If a horizontal incision is encountered over a favored approach site, this should be crossed at an angle greater than 40° to prevent ischemic necrosis of skin edges.

Hardware removal

The majority of femoral osteotomies are secured with internal fixation. In the previously cited series of 215 hips, 211 were fixed with internal hardware, and 72% of patients underwent hardware removal at the time of their arthroplasty.[1] The need for hardware removal at the time of arthroplasty may alter the choice of surgical approach, particularly if a surgeon's preference is normally directly anterior. It can also add to the length of the arthroplasty procedure, thereby incurring added risk for infection. This can be compounded if a surgeon is not prepared to deal with broken hardware or screws that have been stripped. It is wise to have a broken screw set available, as well as burs and potentially trephines, in addition to the appropriate hardware extraction set as identified in previous operative notes. Ferguson and colleagues[1] noted difficulty during hardware removal in 24% and breakage of implants at the time of removal in 21% in his series of 215 hips.

The length of fixation along the femoral shaft may also play a role in implant selection. If all the hardware is to be removed, an implant should be selected that bypasses any residual stress risers created by screw removal. Conversely, a carbide bur may be used to cut a plate short so that only the proximal portion is removed with subsequent implantation of a shorter femoral stem and retention of a portion of distal hardware (**Fig. 1**). The latter technique may allow for a less-extensive soft tissue insult. On rare occasions, removal of the existing hardware incurs such a grievous insult to a patient's soft tissues or bone stock that a hip resurfacing prosthesis proves the most beneficial

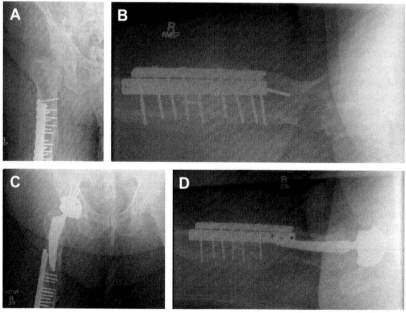

Fig. 1. (*A, B*) Anteroposterior radiographs of a patient with extensive proximal hardware in place. (*C, D*) Postoperative radiographs after THA with short femoral component with hardware retention.

option, because all the femoral hardware may be retained (**Fig. 2**).

Empty screw holes also may increase the rate of intraoperative fracture by serving as a stress riser during femoral preparation. Great care should be taken during rasping, broaching, and reaming under these circumstances. In cases of cemented femoral fixation, empty screw holes may also compromise a surgeon's ability to adequately pressurize the canal. This may lead to a poorer cement mantle and a subsequently increased rate of mechanical failure over time.

A staged approach to hardware removal and THA is another option in the treatment of these patients. Tissue cultures at the time of hardware removal should be obtained routinely. Ferguson and colleagues[1] reported that 28 of 290 patients had positive intraoperative cultures despite absence of any other data to suggest an active infection. If an ongoing infection is detected, it can be treated before THA. Conversely, if tissue cultures are negative, then surgeons are afforded a greater degree of aseptic certainty during subsequent THA.

Abductor mechanism considerations

The position of the greater trochanter is often altered significantly after a proximal femoral osteotomy. If the resultant position of the trochanter overhangs the entry point to the femoral canal, it can complicate stem insertion. Boos and colleagues[2]

noted a significant increase in the need for trochanteric osteotomy during THA after a proximal femoral osteotomy compared with a primary THA control group. The position of the trochanter also needs to be critically gauged with respect to the final tension of the abductors during trialing and after component insertion. The abductors may be long compared with the offset afforded by the femoral implant, especially in circumstances where a calcar-replacing implant is required. A trochanteric advancement should be considered in these instances to improve hip stability.

Femoral version

Rotational alterations performed during an osteotomy vary the normal version of the proximal femur and may obscure the normal bony landmarks often used by surgeons during stem placement. Evaluating the combined version during component trialing can be used as a surrogate assessment of the femoral version when the cup position and acetabular landmarks are more reliable. Often the femoral component needs to be placed in a position of relative retroversion compared with the modified anatomy observed in the previously osteotomized femur. This can be attempted with standard uncemented implants; however, if stable interference fit cannot be achieved, then a smaller stem can be cemented in relative retroversion to "cheat" the patient's anatomy. Modular uncemented stems,

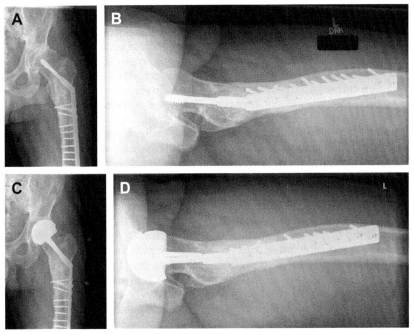

Fig. 2. (*A, B*) Radiographs of a 31-year-old man with fibrous dysplasia and end-stage hip arthritis. Removal of side plate would put femur at risk with fibrous dysplasia. (*C, D*) Postoperative radiographs after resurfacing arthroplasty with hardware retention.

which pair a proximal metaphyseal fitting sleeve and a distal fluted stem, allow for any degree of selected version and are a powerful tool for addressing this deformity. The use of intraoperative radiographs to assess component position is another means of providing feedback to surgeons and helps ensure operative success.

Results

THA after a proximal femoral osteotomy is usually performed in a younger more active population than standard primary THA.[2] In the studies reviewed, the average time from a varus/valgus-producing osteotomy until conversion to a total hip varied from 7.3 to 12.4 years[1–4] in patients with mean ages between 50 and 61 years. Rotational osteotomies had a shorter survivorship and were converted between 1.7 and 4 years in patients with mean ages between 40 and 43 years.[5,6] The higher demand this patient population imposes on their components has affected reported results with early stem designs and implantation techniques. Historical results with cemented stems, using first-generation and second-generation cementation techniques, demonstrated a higher complication rate and a greater degree of procedure difficulty compared with standard primary THA.[1,2] Ferguson and colleagues[1] noted a 19.5% mechanical failure rate of cemented stems, with a 12% stem revision rate at 10-year average follow-up. This series also highlighted a 25% complication rate, technical difficulty in 23% of patients, and an overall aseptic revision rate of 15%. Another study, performed by Boos and colleagues,[2] noted a trend of decreased survivorship (82% vs 90%) in a group of 74 cemented THAs after a proximal femoral osteotomy compared with a control group of 74 cemented standard primary THAs at follow-up between 5 years and 10 years. This series also noted a significant increase in technical demand and longer procedure times in the postosteotomy group. Both of these studies, however, pointed out a significant improvement in hip scores after the THA procedure.

Results of THA after proximal femoral osteotomy improved dramatically with newer implant designs and a shift toward greater reliance on uncemented instrumentation techniques. Breusch and colleagues[3] reported 10-year results of 44 uncemented stems implanted after failed intertrochanteric osteotomy and a 96% survivorship rate when aseptic loosening was selected as the endpoint. They concluded that this was comparable to patients with normal anatomy undergoing a standard primary THA. They noted 2 fissures that occurred during instrumentation, but these did not require any further treatment. Another more recent study investigating 30 uncemented THAs performed

after failed valgus osteotomy in the setting of acetabular dysplasia demonstrated a stem survivorship of 100%.[4] Eleven of these patients received modular stems that allow for version variability, with the remainder receiving monoblock stems (with modular femoral head sizing). The investigators noted cortical hypertrophy at the tip of 6 monoblock stems and concluded that, secondary to this radiographic finding and the ease of addressing version abnormalities, modular stems should be preferentially used in this patient population.

THA after rotational osteotomy has also been evaluated in isolation. Kawasaki and colleagues[5] compared THA after rotational osteotomy for AVN to primary THA for AVN. At midterm follow-up, there were no differences in Harris hip scores, radiographic loosening, or survivorship between groups. In a similar subsequent study by Lee and colleagues[6] comparing postrotational osteotomy THA with standard primary THA, the investigators noted a higher percentage of malpositioned femoral stems with respect to varus/valgus alignment. Acetabular cups in the conversion group were also found to have a greater chance of being underanteverted and underabducted. This study failed to correlate these findings with differences in clinical outcomes, however.

THA AFTER PERIACETABULAR OSTEOTOMY
Technical Pearls

Overview
Periacetabular osteotomies are usually performed in the setting of developmental dysplasia to relieve pain and improve coverage of the femoral head, thereby improving hip mechanics and contact stress placed on the femoral and acetabular cartilage. The characteristic deformity observed in developmental dysplasia of the hip is a shallow, vertical, lateralized, and overanteverted socket. The degree to which these deformities occur, the residual congruency of the hip joint, the condition of the articular cartilage, and patient age direct surgical treatment.

A multitude of osteotomies has been described and a thorough discussion of each is beyond the scope of this article. The focus instead is on THA performed after Salter, Chiari, triple, and Bernese osteotomies. Salter, triple, and Bernese osteotomies are complete and redirect the acetabulum to varying degrees to gain added coverage of the femoral head. Chiari osteotomies are also complete but rely mainly on translation rather than rotation to medialize the acetabulum. They are often subsequently augmented with a slotted shelf procedure to gain the desired femoral coverage. Salter, Chiari, and triple osteotomies are performed in patients with open triradiate cartilage, whereas Bernese osteotomies are reserved for patients who are skeletally mature. Each type of osteotomy that is converted to a THA requires special attention and has its own surgical considerations with respect to incision placement, approach, hardware removal, and cup positioning.

Incision selection and approach

Salter, Chiari, and Bernese osteotomies are routinely performed through an anterior approach using the interval between the sartorius and tensor fasciae latae. A triple osteotomy is usually performed through two incisions: a transverse incision centered over the ischium and a bikini-type iliofemoral incision. The positions of these incisions do not compromise any of the traditional approaches to the hip. Anterior approaches may use the previous incisions, and direct lateral and posterolateral approaches have the luxury of unviolated tissues. Often, however, additional procedures have been performed previously, including proximal femoral osteotomies, which may compromise the desired incisional site (discussed previously). Furthermore, alterations in femoral anatomy from dysplastic sequelae or previous surgery may require a trochanteric osteotomy. Parvizi and colleagues[7] reported a series of 45 Bernese osteotomies converted to THA and noted that a transtrochanteric approach was needed in 24 cases due to associated femoral deformities.

Hardware removal

Salter and triple osteotomies do not leave any permanent hardware that requires removal at the time of conversion to THA, because most are performed in children with temporary percutaneous fixation removed at 8 to 12 weeks. Chiari osteotomies that have been augmented by bone grafting may have several screws supporting the graft. Bernese osteotomies are fixed in place with 3 screws directed from the iliac wing into the mobile segment. In the series by Parvizi and colleagues,[7]

discussed previously, none of the hardware placed during a Bernese osteotomy required removal at conversion to THA. If, however, screw tips are encountered during acetabular reaming, a helicoidal bur may be used to recess the screws to a level below the anticipated bone-implant interface.

Cup positioning and fixation

The considerations with regard to cup position after an osteotomy depend partially on an osteotomy's success in correcting the initial deformity. In cases of developmental dysplasia of the hip, the acetabulum is often lateralized and overanteverted. After a Chiari osteotomy, which works to primarily medialize the cup, there still may be increased anteversion of the acetabulum leading to anterior uncoverage of the component. The same may be the case after Salter osteotomies, which work through decreasing the verticality of the cup but do not adjust the version significantly. On occasion, a Salter osteotomy may markedly retrovert the acetabulum. When placing an acetabular component into a retroverted socket, care must be taken to ensure appropriate anteversion is achieved. In mild cases of acetabular retroversion, placing the socket proud posteriorly with subsequent trimming of the prominent anterior rim serves as an adequate technique to produce the desired version. In instances of significant retroversion, posterolateral bone grafting with native femoral head or a portion of the anterior acetabulum may be required to certify proper osseous support of a properly positioned component. Triple and Bernese osteotomies are able to generate greater correction with respect to acetabular version and THAs placed into these corrected sockets must often account for acquired retroversion and posterior uncoverage. In the aforementioned series of 45 Bernese osteotomies converted to THA, 23 sockets were judged to be in a position of relative retroversion.[7] There were no posterior column deficiencies reported in this series (**Fig. 3**).

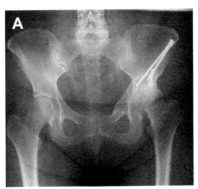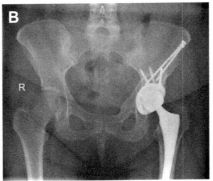

Fig. 3. (*A*) Anteroposterior radiograph of a patient with end-stage hip arthritis 7 years after periacetabular osteotomy. (*B*) Postoperative radiograph after uncemented THA.

Medialization of the socket after previous osteotomy also has implications on component selection and positioning. In a study by Minoda and colleagues,[8] biomechanical parameters of THAs performed after Chiari osteotomies were compared with a control group who did not undergo a prior osteotomy. Converted THAs were found to have a greater vertical joint reactive force angle. The investigators believed this could act to distract rather than compress the acetabular component with joint loading, especially in DeLee and Charnley zone III. Given this concern, additional screw fixation in the ischium during cup placement may be prudent to prevent early loosening or fibrous ingrowth of the component in this zone. The use of high offset stems may also help combat the effects of socket medialization by increasing the horizontal vector component of the joint reactive force and decreasing the abductor force angle.

Results

Tokunaga and colleagues[9] reported the results of THA after failed Salter osteotomies in a mixed series evaluating both Salter and Chiari conversions. In this series of 52 THAs, previous Salter osteotomies were performed in 40 instances and both Salter and Chiari were performed in an additional 3 instances. The average lag between Salter osteotomy and THA was 22.6 years when performed in isolation and 12.7 years when performed in addition to a Chiari osteotomy. There was no difference between the conversion group and a control group of primary THAs with respect to intraoperative fracture rate, dislocation, Harris hip scores, or survivorship with 8-year follow-up.

The results of conversion THA after a failed Chiari osteotomy have also shown encouraging results with short and midterm follow-up. Hashemi-Nejad and colleagues[10] evaluated 28 THAs performed after a failed Chiari osteotomy with an average follow-up of 5 years and compared this cohort with a control group of 50 patients with hip dysplasia who underwent THA without a previous osteotomy. They reported equivalent clinical and radiographic results between groups and a decreased need for bone graft augmentation to achieve adequate acetabular component coverage in the postosteotomy group. They also reported decreased operative time and blood loss in the conversion group. These results differ from those of Minoda and colleagues,[8] who reported an increase in the operative time and blood loss in 10 THAs performed for failed Chiari osteotomy when compared with a group of 20 matched controls. Their study also provided biomechanical analysis, which indicated that a more vertical joint

force resulted in the conversion group and raised concern for the long-term survivorship of acetabular components in this group. The study by Minoda and colleagues had only 3 years of mean follow-up, and at that time clinical and radiographic outcomes were equivalent between experimental and control groups.

Peters and colleagues[11] reported the results of THA conversion of a failed triple innominate osteotomy compared with a group of controls undergoing THA for osteoarthritis with 3-year follow-up using uncemented components. They noted equivalent survivorship, patient function, acetabular coverage, and radiographic results between the groups in their study. Patients in the conversion group, however, had increased residual hip pain postoperatively and decreased Harris hip scores compared with controls. The conversion group also had increased blood loss and incurred a higher technical demand.

The results of THA after a failed Bernese osteotomy have been reported by Parvizi and colleagues[7] but have not been compared with results in a control group. The conversion THA was performed at an average of 6.3 years after the initial periacetabular osteotomy. In this series, 39 of the 45 THAs yielded excellent or good clinical results. One case of aseptic acetabular loosening was identified. The acetabular component used in most (36) cases was a Ganz-type antiprotrusio cage. One dislocation occurred and was thought to arise from a retroverted cup. Heterotopic ossification was noted in 4 hips and only required surgical intervention in 1 hip. Based on these findings, the investigators concluded that a previous Bernese osteotomy does not compromise the results of a subsequent THA but does add some technical demand, especially with regard to cup positioning, recognizing that the acetabulum is commonly retroverted secondary to the previous osteotomy.

REFERENCES

1. Ferguson GM, Cabanela ME, Ilstrup DM. Total hip arthroplasty after failed intertrochanteric osteotomy. J Bone Joint Surg Br 1994;76:252–7.
2. Boos N, Krushell R, Ganz R, et al. Total hip arthroplasty after previous proximal femoral osteotomy. J Bone Joint Surg Br 1997;79:247–53.
3. Breusch SJ, Lukoschek M, Thomsen M, et al. Ten-year results of uncemented hip stems for failed intertrochanteric osteotomy. Arch Orthop Trauma Surg 2005;125:304–9.
4. Suzuki K, Kawachi S, Matsubara M, et al. Cementless total hip replacement after previous intertrochanteric valgus osteotomy for advanced osteoarthritis. J Bone Joint Surg Br 2007;89:1155–7.

5. Kawasaki M, Hasegawa Y, Sakano S, et al. Total hip arthroplasty after failed transtrochanteric rotational osteotomy for avascular necrosis of the femoral head. J Arthroplasty 2005;20:574–9.

6. Lee YK, Ha YC, Kim KC, et al. Total hip arthroplasty after previous transtrochanteric anterior rotational osteotomy for femoral head osteonecrosis. J Arthroplasty 2009;24:1205–9.

7. Parvizi J, Burmeister H, Ganz R. Previous Bernese periacetabular osteotomy does not compromise the results of total hip arthroplasty. Clin Orthop Relat Res 2004;423:118–22.

8. Minoda Y, Kadowaki T, Kim M. Total hip arthroplasty of dysplastic hip after previous Chiari pelvic osteotomy. Arch Orthop Trauma Surg 2006;126:394–400.

9. Tokunaga K, Aslam N, Zdero R, et al. Effect of prior Salter or Chiari osteotomy on THA with developmental hip dysplasia. Clin Orthop Relat Res 2011;469:237–43.

10. Hashemi-Nejad A, Haddad FS, Tong KM, et al. Does Chiari osteotomy compromise subsequent total hip arthroplasty? J Arthroplasty 2002;17:731–9.

11. Peters CL, Beck M, Dunn HK. Total hip arthroplasty in young adults after failed triple innominate osteotomy. J Arthroplasty 2001;16:188–95.

Bearing Surface Considerations for Total Hip Arthroplasty in Young Patients

George J. Haidukewych, MD*, Jeffrey Petrie, MD

KEYWORDS

- Bearing surface • Total hip arthroplasty • Young

KEY POINTS

- Consider the next operation (revisability) of any implant in young, active patients.
- Hard-on-hard bearings have generally not resulted in significantly lower wear and less reoperations (survivorship) in young, active patients. Squeaking, sensitivity to component position, and adverse reactions to debris remain concerning.
- Modern ceramic or metal on modern polyethylenes probably represent the most predictable bearing choices for young, active patients in 2012; however, long-term data are needed to properly support this assumption.

INTRODUCTION

Over the past few decades, various procedures have been introduced to preserve the native hip joint in young patients. Concerns about wear-related premature failure of arthroplasty in young patients remain. Despite our best efforts, in some situations, arthroplasty is the only remaining reasonable reconstructive option. Few patients are willing to accept arthrodesis of the hip when presented with the alternative of hip arthroplasty. Modern advances in uncemented technology have essentially solved the problem of long-term fixation of the acetabular and femoral components. Various studies have documented the long-term durability of various ingrowth surfaces and various stem geometries. The preference of component selection will vary by surgeon, bone quality, and anatomy. Cemented fixation in young active patients has generally fallen out of favor in North America. Most surgeons would choose uncemented components for total hip arthroplasty (THA) in young patients. Practically speaking, therefore, the more challenging decision

making surrounds the choice of bearing surface. The purpose of this article is to review various bearing surface choices, their pros and cons, and to summarize the available published long-term data on the performance of various bearing couples, specifically in patients aged younger than age 50.

COMPONENT SELECTION IN YOUNG PATIENTS

When a THA is implanted in a young patient, it is safe to assume that the most likely long-term problem that patient will face in the future is osteolysis from bearing-related wear debris. Every arthroplasty will eventually fail and require revision. With this in mind, it is important, in the authors' opinion, to consider the revisability of any implanted components. For example, a modular, uncemented, acetabular component offers the ease of later liner exchange. Future improvements in bearing surface (ie, next-generation polyethylenes) may be available to further improve the durability of the construct. Such an option is not available

Disclosures: Dr Haidukewych: Depuy (royalty), Synthes and Smith and Nephew (consulting); Dr Petrie: none.
Level One Orthopedics, Orlando Regional Medical Center, 1222 South Orange Avenue, Orlando, FL 32809, USA
* Corresponding author.
E-mail address: docgjh@aol.com

Orthop Clin N Am 43 (2012) 395–402
doi:10.1016/j.ocl.2012.05.008
0030-5898/12/$ – see front matter © 2012 Elsevier Inc. All rights reserved.

Table 1
Summary of published data on various bearing couples in patients aged younger than 50 years

Reference	Bearing Surface	Number of Patients	Mean Age	Mean Follow-Up (mo)	Survivorship
Mont et al,[1] 1993	Metal on PE Uncemented	42	36	54.0	1 revision because of aseptic loosening (2%)
Berger et al,[2] 1997	Metal on PE Uncemented	57	37	106.0	98.8% survivorship at 10 y (acetabular component only)
Dowdy et al,[3] 1997	Metal on PE Uncemented	36	42	63.6	3 of 41 hips (7.3%) revised because of aseptic loosening or osteolysis of acetabular component No revisions for femoral component
Kronick et al,[4] 1997	Metal on PE Uncemented	154	37.6	99.6	2 (1.2%) femoral revisions 5 (3.4%) acetabular revisions for failure
McLaughlin and Lee,[5] 2000	Metal on PE Uncemented	82	37	122.4	No femoral component required revision for aseptic loosening 98% chance of survival of femoral component at 12 y
McLaughlin and Lee,[6] 2011	Metal on PE Uncemented	79	36	192.0	Survival of femoral component (revision for aseptic loosening as endpoint) was 100% at 18 y Survival of femoral component (revision for any reason as endpoint) was 97% at 18 y
D'Antonio et al,[7] 1997	Metal on PE Uncemented (hydroxyapatite)	136	38.4	81.6	No stem revised for aseptic loosening and femoral component mechanical failure rate was 0%
Chiu et al,[8] 2001	Metal on PE Uncemented	45	33	91.2	98% survivorship at 5 and 10 y (revision for aseptic loosening as endpoint)
Capello et al,[9] 2003	Metal on PE Uncemented (hydroxyapatite)	91	39	135.0	Femoral component showed 99.1% survivorship at minimum follow-up of 10 y (1 stem revised because of aseptic loosening)
Singh et al,[10] 2004	Metal on PE Ceramic on PE Cemented and uncemented cups	33	42	120.0	Uncemented stem 100% at 12 y Uncemented cup 96% at 10 y Cemented cup 90.5% at 12 y
Hartley et al,[11] 2000	Metal on PE Uncemented	39	31	112.0	12.5% required revision for osteolysis and PE wear (none because of femoral side)
Dunkley et al,[12] 2000	Metal on PE Uncemented	50	41	84.0	No acetabular components revised for loosening 10.9% acetabular liners replaced for excessive PE wear
Duffy et al,[13] 2001	Metal on PE Uncemented	72	32	123.6	Estimated survival-free revision for aseptic loosening or osteolysis 97.5% (5 y) and 80.1% (10 y)

Study	Bearing	No.	Age	Follow-up (mo)	Results
Crowther et al,[14] 2002	Metal on PE Uncemented	44	37	132.0	98% survival of acetabular component at 10 y; Average wear rate: 0.15 mm/y
Kim et al,[15] 2003	Metal on PE Uncemented	80	46.8	117.6	No aseptic loosening at latest follow-up; 10-y survival with revision as endpoint is 99% for acetabular and femoral components; With loosening as endpoint, 10-y survival is 100%; Average wear rate: 0.12 mm/y
McAuley et al,[16] 2004	Metal on PE Uncemented	488	40	83.0	Survivorship of THA (with revision of cup or stem excluding PE exchange as endpoint): 98.4% (5 y), 93.2% (10 y), 79.0% (15 y); Survival of stem (any stem revision as endpoint): 99.0% (5 y), 98.2% (10 y), 95.0% (15 y); Survival of cup (any cup revision as endpoint): 97.4% (5 y), 87.6% (10 y), 53.8% (15 y)
Kearns et al,[17] 2006	Metal on PE Uncemented	221	41.1	100.8	Overall survival: 81.2% (10 y) and 46.8% (15 y); 21 revisions (30% of all revisions) because of aseptic loosening; Femoral stem survival: 99.3% (5 y), 98.9% (10 y), 96.8% (15 y); Acetabular survival: 98.7% (5 y), 84.6% (10 y), 52.5% (15 y)
Collis,[18] 1991	Metal on PE Cemented	25	<50	178.8	15-y survival rate (need for revision as endpoint) 69%
Barrack et al,[19] 1992	Metal on PE Cemented	44	40.9	144.0	No femoral component revised for aseptic loosening; 11 (22%) cemented acetabular components revised for aseptic loosening
Joshi et al,[20] 1993	Metal on PE Cemented	103	32	192.0	Probability of implant survival at 20 y was 75%; Overall probability of cup survival at 20 y was 84%; Overall probability of femoral component survival at 20 y was 86%
Ballard et al,[21] 1994	Metal on PE Cemented	36	41	132.0	With aseptic loosening that would lead to revision as endpoint, 10-y survival was 83% for acetabular component and 95% for femoral component; 10 hips revised (all because of aseptic loosening of acetabular component): femoral component loose in 2 of the 10
Devitt et al,[22] 1997	Metal on PE Cemented	77	42	217.2	27 hips revised (20.4%): 77% of revisions because of aseptic loosening; Overall probability of implant survival at 20 y 75%
Sullivan et al,[23] 1994	Metal on PE Cemented	57	42	216.0	13% revision rate for aseptic loosening of acetabular component; 2% revision rate for aseptic loosening of femoral component; 22-y survival (revision because of aseptic failure) of acetabular component 76%; 22-y survival (revision because of aseptic failure of femoral component) of femoral component 92%

(continued on next page)

Table 1
(continued)

Reference	Bearing Surface	Number of Patients	Mean Age	Mean Follow-Up (mo)	Survivorship
Smith et al,[24] 2000	Metal on PE Cemented	40	41	190.8	Survival at 18 y (revision for aseptic loosening as endpoint) was 71% for acetabular component and 95% for femoral component
Dorr et al,[25] 1994	Metal on PE Cemented	39	31	194.4	33 of 49 hips revised for aseptic failure (67%) Revision rates: 12% (4.5 y), 33% (9.2 y), and 67% (16.2 y)
Torchia et al,[26] 1996	Metal on PE Cemented	50	17	151.2	29 of 63 hips (46%) failed Failure rate 27% at 10 y, 45% at 15 y
Mulroy and Harris,[27] 1997	Metal on PE Cemented	40	41	183.6	Revision rate for aseptic loosening of femoral component 2% (1 of 51) 10 of 47 (21%) acetabular components were revised for aseptic loosening
Callaghan et al,[28] 1998	Metal on PE Cemented	69	42	279.6	21 of 93 hips (23%) revised because of aseptic loosening (27 total revisions) 18 acetabular components (19%) and 5 (5%) femoral components revised because of aseptic loosening
Keener et al,[29] 2003	Metal on PE Cemented	43	<50	300.0	Survivorship with revision of either component because of aseptic loosening as endpoint at 30 y was 69% Survivorship at 30 y (revision because of aseptic loosening as endpoint) of acetabular component was 72% Survivorship at 30 y (revision because of aseptic loosening as endpoint) of femoral component was 93%
Burston et al,[30] 2010	Metal on PE Cemented	47	39	144.0	10 hips (19%) required revision for mechanical failure of acetabular component Survivorship of cup (revision of cup for cup failure as endpoint) was 81.1% at average of 12 y Survivorship of stem (aseptic loosening or osteolysis as endpoint) was 100% at average of 12 y
Kerboull et al,[31] 2004	Metal on PE Cemented	222	40.1	174.0	Cumulative survivorship at 20 y was 85.4% Survival at 20 years with radiologic definite or probable aseptic loosening as endpoint was 94.8% for acetabular component and 93.1% for femoral component
Fye et al,[32] 1998	Ceramic on ceramic Ceramic on PE Uncemented	58	37	84.0	Probability of survival (revision as endpoint) for series was 96.9% at 11 y Mechanical failure rate was 7.6% for cups and 6% for stems Revision rate was 1.5% for cups and 1.5% for stems

Study	Bearing / Fixation	N	Age	Follow-up (mo)	Outcomes
Sedel et al,[33] 1994	Ceramic on ceramic / Cemented uncemented	113	41	63.0	96% femoral component survival at 10 y; 90.3% acetabular component survival at 10 y
Bizot et al,[34] 2000	Ceramic on ceramic / Cemented uncemented	104	32.3	92.4	9.3% required revision for acetabular aseptic loosening; Survival rates at 10 and 15 y were 84.6% and 80% (revision for mechanical failure as endpoint); Survival rates of femoral component at 10 and 15 y were 94.8% and 84.8%
Ha et al,[35] 2007	Ceramic on ceramic / Uncemented	64	37	66.0	No acetabular or femoral components revised at latest follow-up; Wear of ceramic components was undetectable
Fenollosa et al,[36] 2000	Ceramic on ceramic / Uncemented, cemented, and hybrid	74	38.1	111.6	Survival at 177 mo; Cemented: 80%; Hybrid: 45%; Cementless: 95.74%
Baek and Kim,[37] 2008	Ceramic on ceramic / Uncemented	60	39.1	85.2	No hips showed evidence of aseptic loosening; No hips revised for any reason
Finkbone et al,[38] 2012	Ceramic on ceramic / Uncemented (2 cemented stems)	19	16.4	52.0	1 revision for loose acetabular component 96% survival (revision any reason as endpoint) No ceramic implant fractures
Migaud et al,[39] 2011	Metal on metal / Ceramic on PE	78	<50	151.0	No hips revised in metal-on metal group; 12-y survival (revision as endpoint) was 100%; 11 (28%) hips revised in ceramic-PE group because of wear or osteolysis; 12-y survival (revision as endpoint) 70%
Delaunay et al,[40] 2008	Metal on metal / Uncemented	73	40.7	87.6	10-y survival (revision as endpoint) was 100% 10-y survival (reoperation for any cause) was 96.4%
Kim et al,[41] 2004	Metal on metal / Uncemented	60	37	84.0	No femoral or acetabular component revised because of aseptic loosening
Girard et al,[42] 2010	Metal on metal / Uncemented	34	25	108.0	1 of 47 hips (2.1%) revised for acetabular osteolysis; Survival rate of femoral component at 10 y 100%; Combined survival at 10 y 94.5%
Hwang et al,[43] 2011	Metal on metal / Uncemented	70	39.8	148.8	Survivorship at average of 12.4 y (revision for any reason as endpoint) was 98.7%; 2 hips (2.5%) had a progressive osteolytic lesion; 1 hip revised because of osteolysis possibly secondary to hypersensitivity

Abbreviation: PE, polyethylene.

on a monoblock, all-metal, acetabular component designed to articulate with a large metal head. Many studies support such lesional treatment of osteolytic defects with retention of well-fixed acetabular components. Additionally, modularity offers the insertion of liners with various lipped elevations and offsets and various head sizes to optimize hip stability. Such a need to plan for the future revision is important in patients aged younger than 50 years.

The recent problems with metal-on-metal bearings have caused some concern among surgeons that considered such monoblock, large-head, metal-on-metal articulations as a potential benefit for young, active patients. There is a growing body of knowledge on adverse reactions to metal-on-metal devices, and the true scope of the problem has not yet been defined. Many of these constructs used monoblock, screwless, uncemented, acetabular components that essentially require the revision of a well-fixed cup (with associated bone loss) to perform a bearing exchange. This example has led the authors to abandon any monoblock, single-bearing acetabular components. The authors routinely choose modular, uncemented, acetabular components, which facilitate later bearing exchange and allow multiple bearing options.

HARD-ON-HARD BEARINGS

Theoretically, these bearings offered the potential benefit of low wear rates and potentially lower rates of clinically problematic osteolysis. Ceramic-on-ceramic and metal-on-metal bearings enjoyed periods of popularity in the last few decades. Unfortunately, further follow-up demonstrated that these surfaces were sensitive to component positioning. For example, a slightly vertical cup placement could cause stripe wear and increased debris generation. Ceramic-on-ceramic bearings also occasionally demonstrated the unique but uncommon problem of squeaking. Good results have been reported, but a clear clinical benefit (ie, lower revision rate) has not been demonstrated to date.

Metal-on-metal bearings offered the potential benefit of large femoral head diameters that would optimize range of motion and hip stability. Additionally, the initial impressions were that debris from these bearing couples would be ionic and, therefore, cleared by the kidneys, potentially minimizing the local tissue response to wear debris. Obviously, recent data have demonstrated a concerning rate of local tissue reactions to metal wear debris. Pseudotumors and painful fluid collections continue to occur. The true scope of the problem has not yet been elucidated. The previous concerns have led many North American surgeons to abandon hard-on-hard bearings. It is important to realize that data exist that document reasonable survivorship of metal-on-metal and ceramic-on-ceramic bearings. All designs are not alike, making direct comparisons nearly impossible.

CERAMIC-ON-POLYETHYLENE BEARINGS

Reasonable data exist to demonstrate improved wear performance of ceramic-on-polyethylene bearings when compared with metal-on-polyethylene bearings; however, a clear clinical benefit to these decreased wear rates (ie, greater survivorship) has not been clearly documented. Advances in modern ceramic heads have decreased but not eliminated concerns about fracture, even in young, active patients. Many surgeons currently consider ceramic-on-cross-linked polyethylene bearings as the bearings of choice for young, active patients; however, considerable controversy still exists. Only longer-term follow-up will provide further information on the best bearing choice.

NEWER-GENERATION POLYETHYLENES

An ever-increasing body of data continues to support the improved performance of cross-linked polyethylenes with modern sterilization and packaging processes. The wear rates have improved based on penetration studies; generally, revisions for osteolysis with a modern bearing are rare in the absence of cup malposition. Again, a clear increase in survivorship has not been demonstrated; however, it is probably reasonable to assume that improved wear rates will translate into lower rates of revision for osteolysis. Various manufacturers are adding antioxidant additives to minimize in vivo oxidation. Long-term data supporting this improvement are not yet available. The clinical performance of these newer polyethylenes has also driven surgeons back to polyethylene and away from hard-on-hard bearing couples. Polyethylene liners also offer various offsets, head-size options, and elevated lips that cannot be used in hard-on-hard bearings. Reasonably large femoral heads can now safely be used with modern polyethylenes with a low reported rate of liner fractures. It is clear that metal- or ceramic-on-polyethylene bearings will generate debris and eventually lead to osteolysis; however, this is a problem that can effectively be treated with bearing exchange with or without grafting of osteolytic lesions. Essentially, we know how these bearing couples will fail and how to treat them when they do. The same cannot be said for wear-related problems with hard-on-hard bearing couples.

PUBLISHED DATA

The available data are heterogeneous, with various femoral and acetabular components, various approaches, and multiple surgeons involved. **Table 1** summarizes published data on THA in young patients and delineates the bearing type and survivorship results. Keep in mind that this data cover many decades, and improvements in bearing couples may not allow extrapolation of older gamma-in-air sterilized polyethylene results to the expected performance of modern polyethylenes. It is nearly impossible to make any direct comparisons from the available literature. It is possible, however, to evaluate the larger studies, with contemporary implants and modern sterilization techniques, and to discern some trends in bearing performance. Prospective randomized studies with modern bearings and reasonable lengths of follow-up (at least 15 years) are not available to allow the surgeon to determine which bearing surface is best for a particular patient. A good understanding of the pros and cons of every bearing couple is important, therefore, to guide patients and surgeons alike.

AUTHORS PREFERRED BEARING CHOICE

The authors prefer to use uncemented components, typically a tapered collarless femoral component to load the femur as proximally as possible, and a modular hemispherical acetabular component. These components allow various bearing options and the option of the simplicity of bearing exchange in the future. Typically, a ceramic-on-polyethylene bearing is chosen. Annual radiographs are obtained and scrutinized for wear-related osteolysis. A priority is placed on considering the revisability of any constructs implanted in young, active patients.

REFERENCES

1. Mont MA, Maar DC, Krackow KA, et al. Total hip replacement without cement for non-inflammatory osteoarthrosis in patients who are less than forty-five years old. J Bone Joint Surg Am 1993;75:740–51.
2. Berger RA, Jacobs JJ, Quigley LR, et al. Primary cementless acetabular reconstruction in patients younger than 50 years old: 7- to 11-year results. Clin Orthop Relat Res 1997;344:216–26.
3. Dowdy PA, Rorabeck CH, Bourne RB. Uncemented total hip arthroplasty in patients 50 years of age or younger. J Arthroplasty 1997;12:853–62.
4. Kronick JL, Barba ML, Praprosky WG. Extensively coated femoral components in young patients. Clin Orthop 1997;344:263–74.
5. McLaughlin JR, Lee KR. Total hip arthroplasty in young patients. 8- to 13-year results using an uncemented stem. Clin Orthop 2000;373:153–63.
6. McLaughlin JR, Lee KR. Total hip arthroplasty with an uncemented tapered femoral component in patients younger than 50 years. J Arthroplasty 2011;26:9–15.
7. D'Antonio JA, Capello WN, Manley MT, et al. Hydroxyapatite coated implants. Total hip arthroplasty in the young patient and patients with avascular necrosis. Clin Orthop 1997;344:124–38.
8. Chiu KY, Tang WM, Ng TP, et al. Cementless total hip arthroplasty in young Chinese patients: a comparison of 2 different prostheses. J Arthroplasty 2001; 16:863–70.
9. Capello WN, D'Antonio JA, Feinberg JR, et al. Tenyear results with hydroxyapatite-coated total hip femoral components in patients less than fifty years old: a concise follow-up of a previous report. J Bone Joint Surg Am 2003;85:885–9.
10. Singh S, Trikha SP, Edge AJ. Hydroxyapatite ceramic-coated femoral stems in young patients: a prospective ten-year study. J Bone Joint Surg Br 2004;86:1118–23.
11. Hartley WT, McAuley JP, Culpepper WJ, et al. Osteonecrosis of the femoral head treated with cementless total hip arthroplasty. J Bone Joint Surg Am 2000;82:1408–13.
12. Dunkley AB, Eldridge JD, Lee MB, et al. Cementless acetabular replacement in the young: a 5- to 10-year prospective study. Clin Orthop 2000;376:149–55.
13. Duffy GP, Berry DJ, Rowland C, et al. Primary uncemented total hip arthroplasty in patients <40 years old: 10- to 14-year results using first-generation proximally porous-coated implants. J Arthroplasty 2001;16(8 Suppl 1):140–4.
14. Crowther JD, Lachiewicz PF. Survival and polyethylene wear of porous-coated acetabular components in patients less than fifty years old: results at nine to fourteen years. J Bone Joint Surg Am 2002; 84:729–35.
15. Kim YH, Oh SH, Kim JS. Primary total hip arthroplasty with a second-generation cementless total hip prosthesis in patients younger than fifty years of age. J Bone Joint Surg Am 2003;85: 109–14.
16. McAuley JP, Szuszczewicz ES, Young A, et al. Total hip arthroplasty in patients 50 years and younger. Clin Orthop 2004;418:119–25.
17. Kearns SR, Jamal B, Rorabeck CH, et al. Factors affecting survival of uncemented total hip arthroplasty in patients 50 years or younger. Clin Orthop 2006;453: 103–9.
18. Collis DK. Long-term (twelve to eighteen-year) followup of cemented total hip replacements in patients

who were less than fifty years old. A follow-up note. J Bone Joint Surg Am 1991;73:593–7.

19. Barrack RL, Mulroy RD Jr, Harris WH. Improved cementing techniques and femoral component loosening in young patients with hip arthroplasty. A 12-year radiographic review. J Bone Joint Surg Br 1992;74:385–9.

20. Joshi AB, Porter ML, Trail IA, et al. Long-term results of Charnley low-friction arthroplasty in young patients. J Bone Joint Surg Br 1993;75:616–23.

21. Ballard WT, Callaghan JJ, Sullivan PM, et al. The results of improved cementing techniques for total hip arthroplasty in patients less than fifty years old. A ten-year follow-up study. J Bone Joint Surg Am 1994;76:959–64.

22. Devitt A, O'Sullivan T, Quinlan W. 16- to 25-year follow-up study of cemented arthroplasty of the hip in patients aged 50 years or younger. J Arthroplasty 1997;12:479–89.

23. Sullivan PM, MacKenzie JR, Callaghan JJ, et al. Total hip arthroplasty with cement in patients who are less than fifty years old. A sixteen to twenty-two-year follow-up study. J Bone Joint Surg Am 1994;76:863–9.

24. Smith SE, Estok DM 2nd, Harris WH. 20-year experience with cemented primary and conversion total hip arthroplasty using so-called second-generation cementing techniques in patients aged 50 years or younger. J Arthroplasty 2000;15: 263–73.

25. Dorr LD, Kane TJ 3rd, Conaty JP. Long-term results of cemented total hip arthroplasty in patients 45 years old or younger. A 16-year follow-up study. J Arthroplasty 1994;9:453–6.

26. Torchia ME, Klassen RA, Bianco AJ. Total hip arthroplasty with cement in patients less than twenty years old. Long-term results. J Bone Joint Surg Am 1996; 78:995–1003.

27. Mulroy WF, Harris WH. Acetabular and femoral fixation 15 years after cemented total hip surgery. Clin Orthop 1997;337:118–28.

28. Callaghan JJ, Forest EE, Olejniczak JP, et al. Charnley total hip arthroplasty in patients less than fifty years old. A twenty to twenty-five-year follow-up note. J Bone Joint Surg Am 1998;80:704–14.

29. Keener JD, Callaghan JJ, Goetz DD, et al. Twenty-five-year results after Charnley total hip arthroplasty in patients less than fifty years old: a concise follow-up of a previous report. J Bone Joint Surg Am 2003;85: 1066–72.

30. Burston BJ, Yates PJ, Hook S, et al. Cemented polished tapered stems in patients less than 50 years

of age: a minimum 10-year follow-up. J Arthroplasty 2010;25:692–9.

31. Kerboull L, Hamadouche M, Courpied JP, et al. Long-term results of Charnley-Kerboull hip arthroplasty in patients younger than 50 years. Clin Orthop 2004;418:112–8.

32. Fye MA, Huo MH, Zatorski LE, et al. Total hip arthroplasty performed without cement in patients with femoral head osteonecrosis who are less than 50 years old. J Arthroplasty 1998;13:876–81.

33. Sedel L, Nizard RS, Kerboull L, et al. Alumina-alumina hip replacement in patients younger than 50 years old. Clin Orthop 1994;298:175–83.

34. Bizot P, Banallec L, Sedel L, et al. Alumina-on-alumina total hip prostheses in patients 40 years of age or younger. Clin Orthop 2000;379:68–76.

35. Ha YC, Koo KH, Jeong ST, et al. Cementless alumina-on-alumina total hip arthroplasty in patients younger than 50 years: a 5-year minimum follow-up study. J Arthroplasty 2007;22:184–8.

36. Fenollosa J, Seminario P, Montijano C. Ceramic hip prostheses in young patients: a retrospective study of 74 patients. Clin Orthop 2000;379:55–67.

37. Baek SH, Kim SY. Cementless total hip arthroplasty with alumina bearings in patients younger than fifty with femoral head osteonecrosis. J Bone Joint Surg Am 2008;90:1314–20.

38. Finkbone PR, Severson EP, Cabanela ME, et al. Ceramic-on-ceramic total hip arthroplasty in patients younger than 20 years. J Arthroplasty 2012;27:213–9.

39. Migaud H, Putman S, Krantz N, et al. Cementless metal-on-metal versus ceramic-on-polyethylene hip arthroplasty in patients less than fifty years of age: a comparative study with twelve to fourteen-year follow-up. J Bone Joint Surg Am 2011;93(Suppl 2): 137–42.

40. Delaunay CP, Bonnomet F, Clavert P, et al. THA using metal-on-metal articulation in active patients younger than 50 years. Clin Orthop 2008;466:340–6.

41. Kim SY, Kyung HS, Ihn JC, et al. Cementless Metasul metal-on-metal total hip arthroplasty in patients less than fifty years old. J Bone Joint Surg Am 2004;86:2475–81.

42. Girard J, Bocquet D, Autissier G, et al. Metal-on-metal hip arthroplasty in patients thirty years of age or younger. J Bone Joint Surg Am 2010;92: 2419–26.

43. Hwang KT, Kim YH, Kim YS, et al. Cementless total hip arthroplasty with a metal-on-metal bearing in patients younger than 50 years. J Arthroplasty 2011;26:1481–7.

Index

Note: Page numbers of article titles are in **boldface** type.

Orthop Clin N Am 43 (2012) 403–408
http://dx.doi.org/10.1016/S0030-5898(12)00051-X
0030-5898/12/$ – see front matter © 2012 Elsevier Inc. All rights reserved.

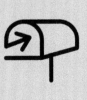
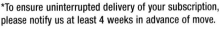

Printed and bound by CPI Group (UK) Ltd, Croydon, CR0 4YY

03/10/2024

01040350-0008